# The TOXIC Labyrinth

**A family's successful battle against environmental illness**

**Myrna Millar, B.Ed, M.B.A. • Heather Millar, B.S.N., R.N.**

**Foreword by Sherry Rogers, M.D.**

**◆NICO◆**
PROFESSIONAL
SERVICES

NICO PROFESSIONAL SERVICES LTD.
VANCOUVER, CANADA

NICO Professional Services Ltd.
1515 West 2nd Avenue  Suite 543
Vancouver BC V6J 5C5
Canada
Phone:  (604) 733-6530
Fax:    (604) 733-6506

Printed in Canada by Hignell Printing Limited, Winnipeg MB
Text printed with vegetable based ink.


**Canadian Cataloguing in Publication Data**

Millar, Myrna, 1940-
         The toxic labyrinth


ISBN 0-9699245-0-X

1. Millar, Heather, 1963- 2. Environmentally induced diseases--
Patients--Biography. 3. Allergy--Patients--Biography. I. Millar,
Heather, 1963- II. Title.
RC585.M54 1995      362.1'96970092      C95-910356-2

This book is dedicated to our fathers.

Dr. William Nikiforuk
'Always listen to the patient.'

and

Norman Millar
"Live life to the fullest.'

and

To the Children
For They are the Future

# ACKNOWLEDGMENTS

## OUR SPECIAL THANKS TO

Two very special people in our lives, Don and Doug, who provided support and counseling throughout a very difficult year and in the writing of this book.

Those health professionals who believed in Heather and whose assistance was crucial to her recovery.

Friends and relatives who gave us their good wishes during this time of crisis and never stopped believing that Heather was truly ill and had the determination and fight to conquer what appeared to be an insurmountable hurdle.

The pioneers who have paved the way in the field of the environment and environmental medicine. Without their information to guide us, we may never have found the way. A number of them are listed in the resources at the back of the book.

Nicole Parton whose article about Heather in *The Vancouver Sun* touched so many people and gave us the inspiration to finish the book.

Cover by Ian Bateson
Cover Photo by Glenn Baglo
with permission from The Vancouver Sun
Copy Editing by Laura Kirk
Authors' photo by Andrew Klaver

# TABLE OF CONTENTS

# FOREWORD

To most people and nearly all physicians, this story may seem like science fiction. But it is a typical story for thousands of my patients from around the world. Although I have never met Heather, I feel I know her intimately, because she presents a similar saga that I and thousands of my patients have lived in part, in whole, and many even beyond this degree of suffering.

Fortunately, we now have many of the biochemical mechanisms and solutions to this 21st Century illness and new data emerges literally, daily. I thank Myrna and Heather Millar for chronicling her story so clearly, for it will help many realize what they have and that they can recover.

For, as Heather and I and thousands of others who have conquered E. I. know, it is primarily through a tremendous amount of knowledge, lovingly imparted, that others may also heal the impossible. We are the first generation of this man-made disease, with bizarre symptoms that totally stump medicine. Understandably, we have all felt the need to share so that we can lessen the burden of others. Thank you Heather and Myrna for a great job.

Sherry Rogers, M.D. 1995

Authors' Note:

Dr. Sherry Rogers is recognized as a foremost authority in environmental medicine. Because environmental illness, regardless of individual symptoms and labels, requires such profound patient education, she has authored a number of books in this field, namely *The Revised E. I Syndrome, Tired or Toxic?, You Are What You Ate, The Cure Is In The Kitchen, Wellness Against All Odds,* and *The Scientific Basis of Environmental Medicine.* Currently, Dr. Rogers is working on three new publications. Because of the information these books provide, many who suffer can realize their goal of wellness less expensively and without leaving home.

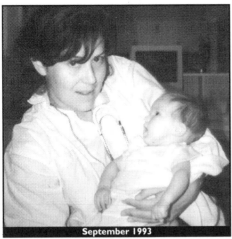

**September 1993**
Into the Labyrinth

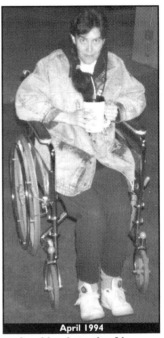

**April 1994**
Looking into the Abyss

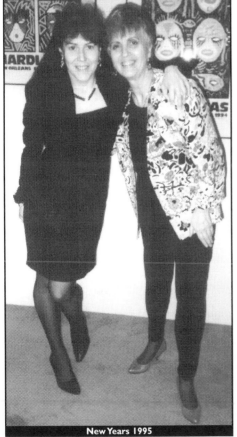

**New Years 1995**
Into the Future

*Heather's*

*Progress*

*Through*

*the*

*Labyrinth*

# IF WE HAD KNOWN THEN WHAT WE KNOW NOW

# The Toxic Labyrinth

I look out my window at the bright morning sun bathing the marina with its September warmth, at the mountains, their peaks shrouded in clouds. Fall heralds the end of an arduous year that has tested the strength and determination of my daughter and those closest to her.

On September 28, 1993, my daughter, Heather, collapsed at work. This episode, we thought, must have a simple solution. As the days became months, our frantic quest for an explanation was fueled by Heather's rapidly declining health. What was causing the continuous weight loss, the constant nausea, the chronic fatigue, the confusion, the myriad of other symptoms, and finally, the inability of her body to tolerate food?

These ongoing assaults on her body were turning a gregarious, fun-loving person into a recluse. This was not the real Heather, well known for her affinity with people and vigorous interest in travel and exploring new places, a dedicated nurse whom many parents had praised for her vitality and effective nursing skills, in making the days of young cancer patients more bearable.

This woman who had embraced life, savoring each moment to the fullest, did not fit the diagnosis of anxiety and stress, which the medical community kept reinforcing each time we sought assistance. Finally, we realized that we had to find the correct path through the maze and challenge an elusive enemy, unaided by conventional medical practice.

What was this insidious enemy that drove us into a labyrinth with indecipherable instructions and only our wits to pit against a sly and wily opponent? We discovered a man made foe disguised in many forms, a force that was able to enter our lives freely, catching us unaware while slowly taking control and holding us ransom. Heather was slowly being poisoned by environmental toxins and she had become allergic to her environment.

Was her condition the result of unusual circumstances, of exposure to a concentrated amount of hazardous chemicals? No, she was living a life style common to the majority of working women.

One, in fact, that was less stressful than most. However, little did she realize her ordinary environment was filled with chemicals that continually bombard the body, a fact that led to her collapse and our subsequent journey of discovery.

So far we have been strong enough and cagey enough to navigate the labyrinth. We have exposed the guile and tactics of our enemy, giving us the power for now to keep the attacking forces at bay. Our determination has enabled us to find a way to escape through the maze and in the process, glimpse at future treachery.

Probing for answers introduced us to many enlightening sources. We read books and articles, spoke to others in similar situations, kept diaries and food logs, made charts, incorporated ancient therapeutic relaxation techniques, and surfed the Internet.

Our observations and findings demonstrate that the toxins in the environment affect each person in different, yet similar ways. This shrewd tactical maneuver by our enemy made it very difficult for us, in the beginning, to unravel the secrets of the labyrinth, because each piece of information we gathered was only one small part of a much larger image.

It would be easy to place blame on the medical community, whose conservative practices are not attuned to the broader picture of our changing world. Despite our frustration, those practitioners we encountered cannot be faulted for lack of knowledge in their specialized fields. Most were competent professionals whose diagnoses, based on available tests, were accurate. However, the practice of medicine has become a profession of compartments and departments. Patients are rarely observed as whole beings who interact within an environment that affects the entire body, not just one of its parts.

In many ways the medical community mirrors what society expects. Many of us would rather rely on a series of test results than the diagnostic ability of the physician. We are programmed to ask for the quick fix, some potion or elixir which will provided rapid recovery or improvement. Few of us have the patience to nurture and develop healthy bodies, which can function under less than ideal circumstances.

However, the medical community is not the only sector of society that does not understand this escalating problem. Most individuals are concerned about the environment, but are unaware of the consequences of our convenient life style. Our family was no different until we had to meet the challenge. Only now do we realize the ever increasing effects of the environment on our health and the debilitating results for those who have succumbed.

As a pediatric nurse, Heather knows the health care system intimately. As she goes through the various stages of her illness, she relates to the experiences of her former patients who had to face the isolation and harsh realities of diagnosis and care in a large medical facility. Observing the system as a patient causes her to question her training and beliefs, but the break from conventional western medical practices is not easy.

Except for those health care professionals who were instrumental in Heather's recovery, we have enumerated the physicians she encountered. Using this format draws attention to the impact our environment is having on the health care system. Many of those who are affected access the system numerous times, often without finding an acceptable explanation for their deteriorating condition.

Our search for answers led us down a number of blind alleys. Meanwhile, frustrated by our inability to find rapid solutions, we were driven by the ticking time bomb of Heather's rapidly declining condition. It took the combined efforts of many individuals, armed with specialized knowledge and problem solving techniques, to discover a logical and reasonable approach that would provide results. The exercise resembled an intense research project, one that yielded information beyond any initial expectations.

# If We Had Known Then What We Know Now

Only after exhaustive searching were we lucky enough to encounter, in person or through published research materials, a few enlightened health care professionals and knowledgeable individuals who are working toward a better understanding of our new world and its power over our health and well being. Through their efforts and our persistence, Heather has slowly regained her health and former vitality. Her recovery, slow as it appeared, was a dramatic improvement considering the place from which she started and measured against others with comparable histories.

By relating Heather's story, we hope to alert you to the inherent dangers from substances we encounter daily. Environmental illness affects each of us differently because of our exposure to these toxic substances and our particular genetic and nutritional backgrounds. These factors make diagnosis and providing specific solutions difficult. Our search for answers and our observations along the way are not offered as scientific facts, rather as information you can use to assess your own life style and state of health. You may want to make some simple changes, now, before increasingly radical changes are forced upon you in the future.

We mention no products, facilities, nor health care professionals by name. Our intent is not to promote any one type of treatment or product, but to show there is assistance available. In the Conclusion, we have designed a checklist to help you assess your own situation. Resource materials and associations which provide guidance and information are listed at the end of the book.

Heather's ordeal is not uncommon. Along the way we have met many people, mostly women, who have similar stories to tell. As her story unfolds, I am certain many of you will find some comparisons to circumstances in your own lives. We are convinced that others need to know of our experiences. This conviction comes from our feeling of helplessness during the illness, one that stemmed from not knowing which way to turn or where to find the answers, while we watched Heather, an active, fun-loving, and bright thirty-one year old, change before our eyes into an emaciated, depressed old woman.

Had we known then what we know now, we could have met the challenges before the actions demanded significant amounts of physical, emotional, and financial resources. Environmental illness appears endless, and for those who do not find a way out, it remains that way. If we can warn one of you or someone in your family to the dangers you may face from the environment, writing the book will have been worth the time and effort.

If we wrote only of findings and observations, you would not come to know the people who struggled so hard. We have, instead, shared our innermost thoughts and feelings. Our story is not a case study, one that dwells only on the physical aspects of a problem, but rather illustrates the loneliness as well as the devastation chronic illness creates on the emotional, social, spiritual, and physical side of the individual.

As we share our story you will identify with us. Why? Because what happened to our family could happen to yours. We are the ordinary people you pass in the supermarket or the mall, your neighbor, your colleague at work.

What follows is Heather's story. It is a story about my daughter, her determination to beat what appeared to be insurmountable odds, the family that stood behind her, and the external forces that have changed our lives.

**CHAPTER 1**

# INTO THE LABYRINTH

The complexity of the maze was not apparent until I had ventured into the first passage.

# The Toxic Labyrinth

## 1993

### September 30

The uneasiness returns shortly after my morning coffee. The aching muscles, joint pains, and nausea that have plagued me for the last couple of days is escalating. A sensation similar to an electrical shock pulses up and down my back. The cycle is starting again.

"Mom." A message of urgency rings in that one word.

"Heather, what's wrong?"

I can hear the concern in her voice, but I can't reply. Am I having a stroke? I try to talk, to utter just one word. No words come. My mind is functioning. It seems to process what's going on around me, yet my body won't do what my mind is commanding it to do. I want to move my arms and reach out for Mom, who is right here beside me. My frozen limbs won't respond. Are they connected to my body?

"Heather, answer me."

"I'm all right now. I don't know what happened."

It has taken a few minutes to regain my power of speech and movement. Did I imagine what just happened? Sometimes the flu produces weird symptoms and reactions. After a few days rest, I'll be back to normal and forget about this incident. There's no use in causing Mom to worry.

Mom and Doug have come from Vancouver to visit me in Memphis, and I have been taking my duties as guide very seriously. So far, we have toured the Shiloh Battleground, Graceland, and the Sun Recording Studio. Unfortunately, this bout with the flu is restricting me, and I'm going to miss today's scheduled activities.

"Heather, we don't have to go sightseeing. You're too ill. I'm very worried about leaving you alone."

"I took the day off work, to rest and get rid of this flu. That's all this is, a bad case of the flu. Your holiday's almost over. Go and have fun. Besides, I've got your cellular number if I get sick again."

As Mom and Doug prepare to leave, I decide to telephone my boyfriend, Don, who's working in Nigeria. After a few minutes' conversation, a crushing tightness encircles my chest. Unable to ignore the intensity of the pain, I abruptly say good-bye. Mom has just walked out the door. I could call her back, but as I struggle to the window, the trunk of the car vanishes around the corner.

The room is staring to reel. I lie down on the couch. The numbness growing in my hands is affecting my ability to grasp; the pain in my chest pounds incessantly, restricting my breathing. Assuring myself that the incident is only a slight asthma attack, I grab my inhaler. The medicine will relieve the pain in my chest. However, sensation and control on my left side is ebbing and leaves the impression of paralysis. I roll off the couch and crawl to the phone, pushing across the floor with the right side of my body. I try to dial Mom's cellular, but I can't focus. Concentrate. Concentrate on dialing. The call won't go through.

"Someone help me!!"

I phone the apartment manager. "I'll call an ambulance for you," she says.

"No, I'm not that sick." I'm afraid the ambulance will be too expensive.

Bits and pieces of thought patterns try to form whole images in my mind. My illness is no more than a simple flu. Now that my life's going so well, I can't die at thirty. Hopefully, I'll wake from this bad dream at any moment.

The crushing pain in my chest has become almost unbearable, and phoning for an ambulance is my only option. I have to leave for the hospital, before I'm too confused to make rational decisions. My situation gives me insight into the life of the elderly, who are often alone, ill, and in need of help. Because a young person is rarely faced with these issues, it's easy to feel invincible.

The paramedics arrive, but their presence doesn't ease my mind. My left side remains numb, and I can't catch my breath. The inhaler is no longer providing relief.

Suddenly, the ambulance doors slam shut. I am inside the labyrinth. How long will I be at the mercy of its secrets?

---

**Events Prior to September 30**

**Back a Month to August**

It had been a very exciting and invigorating weekend for Don and me, camping and white water rafting in the mountains of eastern Tennessee. The wonders of Tennessee were a new experience for us. I was working in the United States as a pediatric nurse on contract, a 'traveler' as they called me at the hospital. Every few months, I would move to a different city and start another hospital contract. In mid August, I had moved to Memphis from San Antonio.

Don's work schedule included a rotation of one month in Nigeria, working thirty days straight, and one month out on rest and relaxation. He could spend his relaxation time wherever I was working. We always looked forward to a delightful month of spontaneous fun, exploring the sights around my most recent location.

On our way back to Memphis, I noticed a strange rash, red and raised, on the left side of my neck. Dismissing the rash as unimportant, I attributed it to the rubbing of my lifejacket or an insect bite.

After the rash had lasted a week, I developed red, hot spots on my lower extremities. The spots were extremely painful when I walked, because the lesions were concentrated on my shins and ankles. Don was extremely alarmed when he saw them, but I reassured him that the condition, erythema nodosum, was associated with a flare up of Crohn's disease.

I was familiar with the lesions. They had first appeared when I had been diagnosed with Crohn's seven years previously. (Crohn's is a bowel disease that usually affects the small intestine. It can flare up anywhere along the gastrointestinal tract, at any time. Neither the cause nor cure are understood. The usual diagnosis follows symptoms of abdominal pain, stool with blood and mucous, frequent diarrhea, inflammation visible on a special bowel x-ray, and a biopsy of the affected intestinal portion. Although the intestine is the target organ, the disease can affect other organs as well.)

Because of my previous experience, I knew the red hot spots would become less painful, fade into bruises, and disappear. I did think it unusual I wasn't having any stomach pains or related problems.

When the bruises emerged two weeks later, they were accompanied by agonizing arthritic-like pains in my left wrist. My wrist throbbed constantly and interfered with my work. One of my primary functions, as a pediatric nurse, was administering medication. It became an effort to open the vials. My wrist pain soon mushroomed into numbness and tingling in the left side of my neck and shoulder. As well, I had difficulty grasping with my left hand.

Mom and Doug had arrived for a visit the last week in September. I was attempting to show them the main tourist sights in Memphis, in addition to working a daily shift from four to twelve. I associated the joint pains with being tired, having a touch of the flu, and trying to cram too much into my day.

**September 28**

The mall, a complex of quaint brick buildings, housed many fashionable boutiques. There had been subtle hints from Don that he was planning to propose. While Mom was in the city, she and I had decided to shop for my wedding dress.

Our excitement rose as we pulled the old-fashioned, creamy lace gown; adorned with seed pearls and pink rosettes, from the rack. We could visualize the ensemble, complete with a wide brimmed hat and cream-colored satin pumps. I could lose a few pounds before the wedding and look stunning.

Hampered by the constant tiredness, pain, and flu-like symptoms, my excitement was less than it should have been. Although I tried to ignore my right leg while we were shopping, it dragged as I walked. To maneuver the curb, I had to lift my leg using my arms.

"Mom, I've been feeling sick since you arrived. I want to show you all the sights in Memphis, but I don't seem to have the energy. I might make a doctor's appointment after you leave."

Later in the day, while I was driving to work, I thought about the reality of my situation. There was something really wrong. Perhaps, what was bothering me was a little more than the flu. As these thoughts were going through my head, I started to lose my grip on the steering wheel, and no matter how hard I tried to hold on to the wheel, I couldn't find the strength in my left hand.

I parked the car in the hospital parking lot and started to cry. Hopefully, my problem was something simple. Working in the health system, I'd heard horrendous stories about medical costs that had escalated into financial ruin. Before starting my shift, I would make a doctor's appointment.

As I walked onto the ward, the waves of illness convinced me I couldn't handle an eight hour shift. Maybe four hours was more reasonable. I started to make the rounds on my patients, passing out the four o'clock medicines. My left arm was leaden. Supporting it with my right hand to obtain some relief, I attempted to hang intravenous (IV) medication on one of the patients, but I didn't have the strength to lift the medicine up to the IV bag. I knew I had to return home as soon as possible. At the nursing station, I charted the initial patient assessments and explained to the charge nurse that I was unwell and would be leaving early.

The wave of severe sickness was unexpected. A sensation of burning pulsated up and down my back. Had someone taken a cattle prod to my back, searing each of my nerves individually and simultaneously? My nerves were on fire. The surges of nausea were overwhelming. I was rapidly becoming confused and disoriented.

I called to Dawn, a co-worker. By the time she reached me, I could see and hear, but my limbs were immobile. Dawn moved me by wheelchair to the emergency room. Because the pediatric hospital where I worked couldn't accommodate adult patients, the emergency room nurse suggested calling an ambulance to take me to an adult facility. When I heard the word 'ambulance', all I could think about was the cost. My condition was improving, since most of the symptoms had dissipated, replaced by a sensation of general malaise, of inebriation. Holding my head erect had become my main preoccupation. Understanding my predicament, Dawn arranged a ride to another hospital.

Slowly, I walked into the emergency room reception area, every movement requiring my total concentration. For the next hour, I gathered all my will power in a effort to sit up. The receptionist, working through the admitting procedure, had no comprehension of the word emergency. What hospital process required over an hour to process the three lonely soles waiting for her attention?

The overwhelming wave of nausea hit, forcing me to walk outside and spare myself the embarrassment of throwing up in the emergency waiting area. (If I had vomited right there, maybe the receptionist would have paid more attention to me.) After gagging and heaving, I began to feel better. I was no longer struggling to hold up my head. For the first time in days, I didn't sense any pain in my left side. There was no reason to hang out in emergency to be ignored.

# The Toxic Labyrinth

The lack of money in my wallet motivated me to maintain my composure, and I was able to hold my head up long enough to manage the thirty-five minute trip home. The interstate route I normally drove was not an option, and I navigated using the local streets. After only one stop, I arrived home and collapsed on the couch, waves of sickness hammering my body. The heaviness in my arm and leg had subsided, but the pain in my left side silently made its presence known, a nasty reminder of the day's events.

That night I was happy to escape into sleep, to find relief for a few hours. I awakened from my restful sleep with a start. The pulsating and burning in my back had returned and my hands and feet felt numb and frozen. Repeatedly, I tried to clench my hands, which were so numb it took all my concentration to command them to move. Within a few minutes, the sensations had subsided, but when I closed my eyes, the pounding of my heart echoed inside my head. Fear was carving out a permanent place in the back of my mind. The same scenario repeated itself twice more during the night. Were these weird symptoms caused by Crohn's disease? Maybe my doctor's appointment in the morning would reveal the answer.

## September 29

Doctor G1, a gastroenterologist, was a specialist in bowel disorders. As he listened intently to my symptoms, he asked about the episodes of confusion and concluded that blood tests and a CT scan of my head should provide answers.

In preparation for the scan, I was going to experience an IV for the first time. It's one thing to start an IV on a patient; it's another to be the patient. Nursing facts ran through my mind. I recalled all the difficulties that could occur with the procedure. What if the IV wasn't started correctly? What if it took six tries to get it started? I had certainly observed these problems in the past. What if the plastic sheath sheared off, circulated to my heart, and killed me? After that absurd thought, I asked myself how many times, during my nursing career, I had actually observed such an occurrence. Of course, the answer was none. Still, I was not truly convinced I would escape even those low odds.

The technician started the IV without a hitch, and I breathed a sigh of relief. He was going to infuse a radioactive dye into my vein to enhance the scan and the radiologist's ability to detect any abnormalities in my brain.

My mind drifted to thoughts of my children. (I always referred to my pediatric patients as my children.) The situation was ironic. How many of my children had I sent for these tests? I had never given the procedure a second thought; couldn't even visualize what went on during the test and now I was about to have my own private tour

The tech secured my head to the table with straps. To guard against any possible movement, he tightened a wide chin band, which was rather uncomfortable and confining, at my jaw. No wonder my children had to be sedated before this test. If an adult experienced discomfort at being strapped down, I could appreciate the fear a little child would undergo.

I was lost in my thoughts when the warmth from the dye hit, making my chest feel tight. I had to vomit! How could I vomit? I was on my back, strapped to a table. I waved frantically to the tech, who came over to assess my situation. He let me sit up, take a breather, retch a few times, and regain my composure. Once the nausea had passed, I was ready to continue, even though the confinement of the table made me nervous. My concern was not about the test, but that I might choke before it was completed.

The dye infusion started again, forcing the sickening warm solution through my veins. The crushing pain in my chest returned. The severe wave of nausea hit with maximum force, leaving panic in its wake. I tried not to vomit. I had to sit up. Flailing my arms at the tech, I signaled my distress. He released the straps. I sat up, grabbing wildly for the closest tray. While I emptied my stomach contents, I made a mental note—in case I was subjected to future tests—that I was allergic to the contrast dye. Before proceeding again, the tech and I made a mutual decision to proceed without using the dye. The radiologist would just have to make do.

One last stop to have my blood drawn. Doctor G1 wanted to eliminate lupus and, from what I knew about this disease, I did not want to think about it as a possible cause. Arm extended and vein exposed, I waited patiently to be stuck. Usually, the person on the other end of the needle was me. Part of my daily hospital routine was extracting blood from children who had cancer, and now I was the patient. The experience should build character and empathy, if nothing else. The lab tech appeared with eleven large tubes she planned to fill with my blood. I consciously escaped into the back of my mind.

Throughout the rest of that day, I battled waves of sickness. Doctor G1 had told me to call if I had any concerns or go to emergency if the episodes persisted. I had not planned to make a solo, dramatic entrance by ambulance, but that was the way that it had worked out.

---

**Back to September 30**

When the ambulance attendant places the oxygen mask on my face, a sense of relief invades my body. It's still a struggle to breathe, but I can depend on the oxygen for assistance. The weakness remains along my left side, and my chest is uncomfortably tight. A dullness seeps over my brain, making concentration laborious. The attendant connects the cardiac monitor, which doesn't help to alleviate my apprehension. My training as an open-heart surgery nurse enables me to read the wave lines. Does the monitor indicate an irregular pattern? Is there cause for alarm?

No room for me except in the hallway. The emergency room hums like a colony of busy ants. Nurses dash about trying to cope with the heavy patient load. Two more spells wrack my body while I wait to be examined.

An overworked nurse quickly takes my pulse, blood pressure, and temperature. She fires a series of questions at me, which become obscured by the fog in my head. I have trouble forming coherent answers, but she's too busy to notice. How strange to view medicine from the other side. Instead of the overburdened nurse, I'm the apprehensive patient.

An orderly grabs the end of the stretcher and wheels me into a small room at a remote end of emergency. Alone and far away from the bustle of main area, I review all the possible diagnoses for my condition. The exercise becomes too frightening and I stop. Ignorance is bliss.

Doctor ER1 is examining me. Enough time has elapsed that my head has cleared, and my left side is no longer numb. These changes have brought some relief. He asks me to describe my illness, and I relate the events of the previous two weeks. He orders blood tests, but no chest x-ray. I can't understand his reasoning as one of my chief complaints is shortness of breath, accompanied by crushing chest pain. Too scared, sick, and tired to care, I lie back on the stretcher and close my eyes.

My mind races as I ask myself, "What's happening to me? How can I reach Mom? How am I going to pay for this visit?"

During the eight long hours, I've spent in solitary confinement, the nursing staff have checked on me twice. Stranded in the furthermost regions of the emergency room for so long and without human contact doesn't make me feel secure. However, my chest pain and shortness of breath are starting to ease, and the feeling has returned to my left side. Although I'm uncomfortable on this stretcher with the back rest propped at a ninety degree angle, I have managed to doze for short periods.

## The Toxic Labyrinth

Doctor ER1 has returned with my test results. Normal, all normal. Diagnosis: 'stress', a diagnosis that doesn't make sense. I have an extremely easy job, my personal life is the best it has ever been, and I take holidays every three months with Don.

I blurt out, "Stress is not a reasonable option." His decision remains unchanged.

A note on my discharge papers indicates I should follow up with a family psychiatrist. I snatch the papers from the nurse's hand and head for the phone to call Mom.

Sitting on the curb outside the emergency, I convert what little energy remains into anger. Not only do I still feel sick, but I've also been insulted. The thick Memphis heat cradles my battered body. Tears well up in my eyes. The day has ended leaving me powerless, unable to find any rational answers.

**CHAPTER 2**

# A CRY FOR HELP

My cry for help is of no use because those who can offer assistance can't hear my voice.

# The Toxic Labyrinth

## October 1

I glance at the clock—3 a.m. Chest pain, numb hands, and shortness of breath have awakened me from a deep sleep. A few puffs from my inhaler doesn't help. What did I do with children who had difficulty breathing? Sitting upright and relaxing the body usually worked. Anything to make the feeling to go away.

"I'm so tired. Let me sleep," I cry out at the darkness.

Each time I doze off for a couple of minutes, my labored breathing jars me back into consciousness. Gasping for breath, I try pacing around the limited space of the living room.

Think of nice things, Heather. Paris! I've never been to Paris. Don and I will sip wine aged to perfection, savor French cuisine at quaint sidewalk cafes, and walk hand in hand down the Champs Elysees. The sights, the sounds of Paris. Will Don propose? He's hinted that our October trip will be a romantic vacation. Three weeks. Just three weeks! I can hardly wait.

Up from the depths come the waves of nausea. I can't deal with any additional assaults by myself. If I wake Mom, she'll sit with me and give me comfort until these symptoms abate.

Side by side we lie on the narrow couch, tired from the ordeal, our minds racing with unanswered questions. The three hours of unrelenting chest pain and shortness of breath have finally eased, and I tell Mom to go back to bed. My body craves uninterrupted rest; exhausted I fall asleep sitting up.

I shuffle into Doctor G1's office leaning heavily on Mom's arm. High-backed chairs beckon my weary body with promises of instant gratification. The other patients, elderly but obviously in less distress, observe me with curious detachment. Can't they see that I don't belong here? I'm young and my body is just betraying me for the moment.

The look on Doctor G1's face demonstrates genuine concern. What's he saying? I can't focus on the conversation. Is Mom taking down all the instructions? I want to lie down, to find relief.

The private hospital, solid and respectable, stands like a beacon of hope for my exhausted body. Because the tests haven't produced a logical solution to the events of the past few days, I've been sent to the source of medical information. I avoid thoughts about the expense.

The young cardiologist breezes into my room, takes a cursory history and orders the first in a series of tests, a chest x-ray and EKG. In addition, my bed companion, strapped intimately to my chest, will be a black box, a device to record any irregularities in my heart rate. Only young people who are very sick have heart problems. Am I in that category? I'll try to avoid thinking about that possibility. Tomorrow should bring some answers.

Mom hugs me and tells me not to worry. She'll return early in the morning.

Alone in my room, I itemize all the horrifying medical diagnoses which could be related to my symptoms. I hate myself for knowing so much. Do those of us who work in the medical field make the worst patients? Well, I'm here to test out the theory.

Doctor N1, the neurologist, has interrupted my TV viewing. Leaning his slim frame against the wall, he listens to my story. Each time I go through this exercise, I search the depths of my memory to uncover any information that may provide an important clue.

The focus of his visit appears to center on my personal life. Am I unhappy? How well do I adjust during the month Don spends in Africa? Didn't Don leave immediately prior to the escalation of my symptoms? I assure him that I'm very happy and, in fact, I'm planning a holiday to Paris and don't have time for sickness and hospitals. I have things to do, friends, plans. He alludes to a connection between my numbness and stress and has ordered tests to verify his theory.

After he leaves I wonder why I have to defend myself. Is it impossible to live a low stress life? Why is it so difficult to convince the doctors that I'm happy?

## The Toxic Labyrinth

I watch with curiosity while the nurse starts the IV. Since I have no problem eating and drinking, I assume the procedure validates my presence in the hospital. Maybe the insurance company doesn't allow in-patient investigative testing. With the heart monitor and IV attached to my body, going to the bathroom presents a challenge.

The events of the last week have happened so swiftly it's difficult to adjust to my new role. I'm supposed to be that nurse who is walking by the doorway. But the image of myself as the patient is slowly becoming reality. While I think about my situation, watching each drip of the salt and sugar solution inch its way down the tube to my wrist, one last wave of sickness washes over me, making a blanket to cover me for the night.

## October 2

The fire has danced up and down the nerves in my back since 2:30 a.m. Now, every object in my room has been itemized and rearranged. Anything to divert my attention from this episode. A tremor forcefully rises from an inner recess of my body and converges on each of my muscles simultaneously.

A lull, the sickness has passed.

"Heather!"

I poke my head from under the covers and squint against the light. A wheelchair, parked at the foot of my bed, is joined to a man who introduces himself as the porter, my escort to the testing room. Even though sleep interests me far more than the prospect of a test, I struggle out of bed, the hospital gown displaying my back end without my consent. Gathering my modesty around me, I climb into the wheelchair. Day two in the hospital. Off to the MRI scanner.

The test appears simple enough. I have to lie immobile on a table, while the scanner photographs my head with no other twists to distract me, such as a dye infusion into my veins.

A coffin-like, cylindrical cage is poised two inches from my face. The first attempt to lie within its walls doesn't go well. When the cage begins moving toward the scanner, I call out, "Stop." My breathing problem is increasing in this prone position, and I have to regain my composure. "Please take the cage off." I sit up and take a couple of deep breaths to alleviate the sensation of claustrophobia. The technician suggests that I'll have more success, if I close my eyes. I decide to eliminate the ear plugs, as well.

As I enter the depths of the scanner, a distant voice announces the length of the test and commands me to remain very still. The reason for the ear plugs becomes immediately apparent, when the concert of jackhammers abuses my unprotected ears. The forty-five minutes stretches into infinity, and the test, a trying experience in the best of health, is not enhanced by my nausea and shortness of breath.

Breakfast, typical hospital fare, appears even less palatable after it has waited for my mid-morning return, but I'm never one to say no to food. Whenever I was sick, Mom would say, 'You won't get better if you don't eat.' Words to reinforce the appetite. It's important to eat heartily, nausea or no nausea.

My spirits are improving. Apparently, my heart is in good condition, so I have been relieved of the heart monitor and only the IV remains connected to my body.

Doctor G1 enters as I'm finishing my eggs. "Did anyone mention the mass we detected on your lung with the chest x-ray?" My mind freezes. Have I heard him correctly? A mass in my lung? Through my bewilderment and disbelief, I hear, ". . . CT scan of the chest tomorrow." A CT scan of my chest? People with lung cancer require CT scans. The familiar terror that has lodged in a back corner of my mind charges into my conscious thoughts.

CANCER! CANCER! CANCER! I watch my tears with detachment as they make symmetrical patterns on the white sheet. I can't have cancer. I'm only thirty years old and I don't smoke. I can't tell Don. He's too far away to help and he worries when he can't be with me. Does this mass explain the pain in my chest and my breathing problems?

Mom's calmness fills the room. She has come to the hospital before visiting hours to be with me. "We can't jump to conclusions until after all the test results are in. Let the doctors finish their testing. I've told your grandmothers and Rhonda that you are in the hospital. There is no reason to alarm them before we know what the mass is."

**October 3**

Parked in the wheelchair, marking time before the CT scan of my chest, I take in all the familiar sights and sounds that should make me feel at home. Hospital jargon, standard uniforms, the smell of disinfectant. But I understand the consequences of this mass in my chest. I've worked with cancer patients for three years. Does my fear invade this room? Do the other patients, immobile in their wheelchairs, staring at nothing, perceive my terror?

How can I be sociable with so much on my mind? I must make the effort; the distraction of company will help pass the time.

Onnie, radiant in her white suit, sits beside my bed, her hands calmly resting in her lap. She has dropped in to visit on her way home from church, where she has said a prayer for my speedy recovery. I think about the kindness of this caring woman, who has known me only a short time through work, yet has taken the time to be with me in person and in prayer. Daryl, a compatriot, sits on the edge of my bed. I had nursed with his sister, Akash, a few years ago in Canada. Daryl had looked me up when he was in New Orleans for a pharmacists' convention. Now by coincidence our jobs have brought us to Memphis. Mom gathers us around my bed for a photo session, Heather holding court from her hospital bed.

**October 4**

The team of doctors managing my care is expanding each day, along with my bill. I have a cardiologist to manage my chest pain, a neurologist to assess the numbness in my left side, a rheumatologist assigned to the spots on my legs and joint pain, an infectious disease specialist to interpret the mass in my chest, and a gastroenterologist to check my gut and orchestrate this burgeoning team.

My body isn't viewed as one entity, one functioning unit, but as a number of independent compartments. Each specialist is interested only in his or her area of expertise. To make matters worse, none of the team members communicates with one another, and I must repeat the same information each time one of them makes the rounds.

The rheumatologist has ordered a bone scan to check for arthritis. Each morning the throbbing in my joints signals the beginning of the day. After about two hours, the pain subsides into a dull and omnipresent aching. Is there any portion of my body that's functioning correctly? At this point, only the right wrist and elbow it seems.

The room is crammed with massive machines and a variety of technical staff. The ubiquitous testing table greets me. One of the techs has just explained that the injection of harmless radioactive dye will enable the team to observe my bones and joints in more detail. Harmless! We obviously have different definitions of the word harmless. He's clothed in bulky gloves that reach past his elbows. The syringe containing the dye is housed inside a thick-walled, metal container. With a practiced movement, he reaches inside the container and draws out the syringe while the steel monstrosity looms over my body emitting a steady hum. This nightmare can't be over soon enough. Good health is not something I'll take for granted in the future.

# The Toxic Labyrinth

The nausea, joint pains, and flu-like feeling have plagued me intermittently throughout the day. Am I getting better, worse, or staying the same? It's hard to analyze.

The CT scan of my chest has exposed a one inch mass in the right lower lung. I'm terrified, but I won't share this information with Don until I'm certain of the prognosis. I remember the time I contracted a twenty-four hour flu. When I threw up, he had his shoes on immediately, insisting that I needed medical attention. He's worried enough with the limited information I've relayed to him. It'll be another month before he returns from Africa.

Suddenly, I miss him more than ever, but I have to be brave. Before this crisis, we were allowed one ten minute telephone call each week. His company has made an exception during my illness. Now we talk every other day on the telephone. Hearing his voice gives me the strength to face what lies before me.

Mom has extended her visit a week to be with me while I'm in the hospital, and the two of us can handle the worrying.

## October 5

My eyes open with a start. An unfamiliar sensation. My breathing has stopped! I clutch my throat and sit up in bed, struggling to breathe as I inhale in hard won gasps.

While the nurse takes my pulse, blood pressure, and temperature, I explain the reason for calling her. All readings are normal. My blood pressure is slightly low. Nothing to cause concern. She shrugs her shoulders and says if I become worse to call her again.

What can I do? I escape to the previous week. Don and I laughed as we talked about our trip to Paris, looked at engagement rings, and planned our future home; Victorian and full of antiques. Life was so simple last week. Each deep, labored breath is followed by tears of frustration for what may never be.

Doctor G1 appears before I'm fully awake. He has ordered an upper GI series. Doctor ID1, the infectious disease doctor, will be paying me a lengthy visit today. He's out the door before my mind can comprehend the day's program.

Upper GI series! How am I going to swallow the awful tasting barium, a chalk mixture, flavored to taste like strawberry? I'm well acquainted with this wonderful delight from my previous bout with Crohn's. My nauseous stomach won't relish this pre-breakfast appetizer on the morning menu.

Room service, in the guise of the now familiar porter, whisks me off to the day's testing events. I'm now attuned to the routine and have reserved a second gown, worn backwards, to cover my backside for these morning adventures.

Although my stomach is queasy, I plug my nose and gulp down the fake, strawberry chalk. The test resembles a carnival ride. I'm strapped to a moving table, which rotates and jostles my body, while the tech pats my stomach with a paddle. All the better to see your intestines, my dear. Each of the four sessions on the table are followed by a thirty minute waiting period in the hall. I conjure up images of steak, hamburgers, and pasta to make the barium go through faster.

The cold, hospital breakfast hails my return from the four hour ritual in the barium suite. Fasting for the whole morning has caused my nausea to vanish, and I devour the food as if it's a gourmet meal.

No more testing for the remainder of the day. Mom and I spend our time together laughing and joking, making light of a traumatic situation. I tease her.

"This is the mother and daughter quality time that we are rarely able to schedule. Isn't it fun to spend your holiday in Memphis touring the medical facilities?"

Mom is so positive. She can always take a stressful situation and find an analytical and practical way to approach the predicament.

"Heather, we are faced with a puzzle. Like any other puzzle, when we have enough information, we'll be able to solve it." To emphasize her comment, Mom searches through the medical text I have borrowed, looking for a likely diagnosis, other than cancer, for the mass in my chest.

Evening, and my first encounter with Doctor ID1. Because I have an extensive travel history, he has been asked to join the team. It's time to expand my history to include more than the past few weeks.

---

When I was a little girl, I traveled with my parents and spent most of my Christmas vacations in Hawaii or Texas. From these childhood experiences, the excitement of new places and new people has become an important part of my life.

My travels, when I was an adult, began with a trip to the Virgin Islands followed, by a tour of Japan. The next year, I left Canada to assume my first six month contract as a traveling nurse. I spent three months in both New Orleans and Orlando, using any free time to visit nearby states and local sights. I returned home briefly and worked a few shifts at my former hospital, before leaving again in May of the following year for a six-month trip through the Pacific region with my girlfriend, Melodie. We traveled through New Zealand, Fiji, Australia, Hong Kong, and Thailand.

On the beach in Fiji, Melodie and I slept in a bure with no doors or windows. I was bitten by an insect, and the bite subsequently became ulcerated and infected. I sought medical attention in Australia when the infection began to limit movement on my left side. The doctor surgically removed the necrotic and rapidly spreading infected tissue. The operation left a gaping hole in my side which took six weeks to heal. Melodie, my travel and nursing companion, would change the special bandages each day, when we continued our travels around Australia. The finished bandage, sealed with an abdominal pad similar to a huge maxi pad, was a work of art. Needless to say, I was not at my most attractive while tanning on the beaches of Sydney.

After leaving Australia, we trekked into the hills of Thailand on an elephant and spent a week living with several hill tribes. I lived in bamboo huts, slept on the floor, ate the local food, and washed in the untreated water. Had I exposed myself to some unusual disease?

My return to Canada lasted only six months. Travel was still a priority in my life, so November found me in New Orleans once again. The experience of living and working in one of the world's most fascinating cities was even more exhilarating than before. Fate took an unusual twist. I met Don. My guardian angel had brought me back to New Orleans to find this wonderful man, an engineer who, like myself, had grown up in a small Canadian town.

I worked in New Orleans for nine months on a pediatric cancer unit before taking a similar contract in San Antonio. By that time, Don had been transferred to Nigeria and was able to spend alternate months with me, wherever I was working. During my stay in San Antonio, we made several trips to different parts of Mexico. On our trip to the Yucatan, we traveled with our own sheets, afraid to sleep directly on the supplied bedding. The hotel didn't furnish toilet seats, only in the luxury rooms. We returned to San Antonio with a stomach affliction that remained with us for three weeks.

The months in San Antonio brought a definite decline in my health. Plagued by asthma from the beginning of my stay, I started using an inhaler to relieve the more distressing attacks.

Last March we traveled to England and Wales. That trip was not enjoyable for me, because the damp, musty buildings made it difficult to breathe. I used my inhaler constantly.

Finally, my traveling feet landed me in Memphis, where I have been living for the past two months. Even this city has added its stamp on my health. At the beginning of September, I cut myself with a lancet while taking blood from a child suspected of having hepatitis. The hospital gave me an injection to boost my immune system. Immediately after going to bed that night, I was agitated and my face started to feel numb. Fearing that I might be having a reaction to the shot, I got out of bed to search for information in one of my nursing texts. Total confusion overtook me, and I wandered around the living room in a complete fog, wondering why I was out of bed. After I had gained control, Don insisted I phone emergency to find out what to do. I was given the assurance that my problem was temporary. For the rest of the night, I remained awake, the feeling of agitation making me want to crawl out of my skin. The pain killer that I took provided no relief.

In the succeeding weeks, I started to experience a severe itchiness to the left side of my head and joint pains. Finally, my escalating symptoms forced me to seek medical attention.

═══════════════════════════════════════════════

What is Doctor ID1 thinking? I have just related several incidents, from my travels and working conditions which could be of interest to him. I have been to many different countries and could have picked up anything. Food, especially discovering and sampling exotic dishes, is one of the more delightful aspects of my life. I have always prided myself on being daring. Has my zest for life and adventure landed me in a hospital bed? Since Doctor ID1 is a man who doesn't jump to conclusions, he'll order a few tests to see what the results show.

The first tests are for mumps and tuberculosis. Because nurses are required to have annual tests for TB, I'm familiar with the procedure. Although my TB tests have never been positive; I have been working in public hospitals, nursing mostly poor, underprivileged children. The ominous mass in my lung could very well be TB.

The nurse and I chat as she administers the injections. Right arm for TB, left arm for mumps. Knowing what to expect, I'm fully relaxed. Besides, I always watch carefully to make certain that the procedure is done correctly. The nurse injects the TB solution into my left forearm. The reaction is instantaneous. Has someone hit my head with a very hard, very heavy object? My ears are ringing, my hearing is muffled, and my left arm is burning. As I start to shake, I reach for the nurse's arm. "I'm feeling very ill." A look of concern crosses her face. She rechecks the label on the syringe and reexamines my arm to see if she has accidentally hit a blood vessel. Nothing is amiss.

The sensation has passed, and I release my grasp on her arm. She sits with me for thirty minutes, taking my vital signs to confirm there are no unusual fluctuations in my pulse or blood pressure that could account for the unexpected reaction. Several times she comments on my pale face and sickly appearance.

After she leaves, I pick up a medical text, checking the symptoms and treatments for many types of diseases. As I flip through it, I look for clues to the cause of my condition. I drift off to sleep with descriptions of strange tropical diseases running through my mind.

## October 6

Gasping for breath, I sit upright and lean forward. The left side of my throat is swollen. The nerves in my back are on fire. My left arm is numb. My face is tingling. Every joint aches. It's 1:45 a.m.

The nurse takes my vital signs. Normal. What do I want her to do? My suspicion is that she would rather not call the doctor at this hour. Can I wait to see if the symptoms subside? Why does she ask *me* what to do? Her indecision is not comforting. I check my own respirations. Twenty-four per minute is normal. What's creating this heaviness in my chest?

I turn on the TV, my mindless diversion to relieve the interminable nights. Never this sick when Mom is with me, I despise the loneliness, a feeling that seems to be taking over my life. My mind continues to churn as I review diseases in my head. Do I really have cancer? I do have a low grade fever. Is a low grade fever one of the signs of a cancerous mass?

The night ticks by, the sickness growing with each passing minute. Concentration is becoming arduous. I blink my eyes. A white haze is slowly obscuring the room. I start to shake. The tremors reach a crescendo as they travel through my body, their intensity generating a coldness that oozes into the depths of my tissues. The shaking leaves as quickly as it has come, removing the sickness and crushing pain in my chest. This episode reminds me of similar situations I have observed in my children. When they had high fevers, they would often start to shake as the fever was breaking.

The clock reads 5 a.m., when I drift off to sleep. Will the day bring some answers or just more tests?

The lab technician pushes the door open with authority. Thirty minutes sleep. Another day is beginning. I count the tubes as she pulls them from her basket. Twenty-three!!

"Are all these tubes for me?"

Yes, she nods. Doctor ID1 has ordered a number of blood tests, some of which are so unusual, she has never heard of them. It had taken her thirty minutes to find them in the manual. What weird tropical diseases can my body be harboring?

"Are you going to draw all the tubes at one time?"

"Yes," she answers.

"Has Doctor ID1 ordered a blood transfusion to sustain me after this ordeal?" My early morning attempt at humor elicits a smile.

I've resumed my sleeping position, but sleep is not to be. The man with my chariot has arrived. Rolling my eyes at the sight of the wheelchair, I ask, "Where are you taking me this morning?" I'm not always informed of the test until the porter arrives.

Mornings always bring aching and stiff joints, but this morning I'm having problems with concentration as well as shortness of breath. The lung function test, which may provide some clues to my shortness of breath, involves another piece of machinery to taunt my unstable condition. I think of all the children with cystic fibrosis I've nursed. In just a few minutes, I'll have a better understanding of what was a weekly procedure for them.

The technician observes the oxygen flow from my lungs into my body. The saturation monitor indicates my level is low, which means she has to obtain a baseline blood gas by taking blood from an artery at my wrist. When the technician injects a freezing agent into my wrist, it goes numb. The room is receding. The crushing in my chest is becoming intolerable. Is my throat closing?

I convey my distress to the technician. Another white-coated figure is recruited into action and aims for the artery at my wrist, while the first tech holds my body in a sitting position. In the background, I hear the alarm on the oxygen saturation monitor ring, indicating that my saturation level is falling lower. I gasp for each breath. An eternity passes before he locates my artery. The needle stabs into the vessel, ricocheting pain deep into my shoulder. The freezing is useless. Am I going to collapse? The now familiar fog is invading the testing room. Objects spin through the fog, whirling faster and faster with each breath. I place my head in front of me on the table to make the spinning stop.

Fifteen minutes has elapsed, and the haze lifts like a curtain at the commencement of a play. My breathing has eased. The saturation monitor has stopped its strident alarm. The technician asks if I want to continue with the test. Although my wrist continues to throb, I consent so I won't have to endure this preparation twice. Despite the fact that my shortness of breath makes it difficult for me to blow into the mouthpiece, the test proceeds without further incident.

Off to nuclear medicine I wheel, so exhausted that sleep is the only thought occupying my mind. Waves of sickness continue to assault me. The solid assistance of the waiting room wall keeps my head erect, while I anticipate the next test. Reclining on the testing table will be a welcome treat.

Another mouthpiece to breathe into. Do they not realize how difficult it is for me to breathe? I watch the staff prepare the scanner. Why has no one explained this procedure to me? Do they expect me to know what a lung scan is, because I'm a nurse? I'm a patient and I want to be treated like one.

As if he has been reading my thoughts, the technician begins to explain the procedure. Once again, I'm going to be injected.

# The Toxic Labyrinth

Injections, injections, and more injections. I'm becoming a human pin cushion. Can't they give me one injection to last the whole day? They could inject me with the wrong solution. It's happened before. The injections with radioactive solutions are additional violations my body doesn't tolerate well. What effect are these intrusions having on my condition?

The test promises to be complex with two technicians rather than one. My lucky day, the one handling the syringe appears to be a student. Visions of the days when I was an uninformed, bumbling student flash through my mind, and I close my eyes hoping for the best. The syringe in the large metal container. The heavy, protective gloves. Am I having deja vu? Despite his trembling hands, the student hits my vein, and the mysterious contents of the syringe become a part of me. What a welcome effect! No reaction! Only the stab of the needle breaking my skin.

The large metal disk hovers over my chest. As I blow into the mouthpiece, tears flow across my checks dripping into my ears. I can't make them stop. What'll I do if the mass is cancerous? I can't bear the thought of chemotherapy. I've watched too much suffering during my career as a nurse to go through that. Lung cancer is so final. Treatment only extends life for a few months. It doesn't cure the disease.

Why is this happening now? Just last week, Don and I had talked about our happiness and the great life we were going to have together. We had started planning our future, marriage, children, a home. It has taken me ten years to find this man and this happiness. Is life playing a cruel joke? More tears fall, but I don't care if the technicians notice. I'm tired of hiding my frustration and fear.

The blackness of the Memphis night knocks at my window, announcing the end of another harrowing day. Bouquets of flowers, get well missives from friends and family, line the sill, their vibrant colors mocking me. How long will I be able to enjoy such simple pleasures?

The lung biopsy, a risky procedure, is scheduled for the morning. Visions of a collapsed lung haunt me. I recall the children under my care with collapsed lungs, chest tubes inserted to re-expand the deflated lung. The rhythm of the bubbling water from the tubes would break the silence of the ward during the night shift.

## October 7

A new strategy. I'll stay awake until after my early morning spell. No point in being awakened out of a sound sleep.

The night nurse comes in promptly at midnight to carry out her first and last check for the night, a routine I find unusual. I had always checked my patients every hour. Most of my problems occur at night, and if I don't require hourly monitoring, I might as well be sleeping at home.

The black and white figures from a quieter, gentler era, pledge undying love as the TV movie reaches its climax. A wave of nausea interrupts their passion. Perfect timing.

Unable to swallow, I start to panic. I try to explain my problem to the nurse while I lean forward to catch my breath. She listens, takes my vital signs, and gives me an ice pack for my throat. My only solace is tears. If only Mom or Don were with me, their presence would bring an element of calm to my chaotic plight. What if I stop breathing? Would these nurses know what to do? On an ear, nose, and throat floor, what do the staff know about lung problems?

The waves of sickness continue to buffet me unmercifully, and the ominous haze has returned to afflict my vision. When I close my eyes, I feel as if a wide collar is tightening around my throat. Gasping, I pray for relief. Finally, the shaking and the chilling cold announce that peace is on its way.

Biopsy day. Day of terror. The hubbub of breakfast service gives notice that the porter will appear shortly.

Yesterday, the doctor performing the biopsy spent time with me explaining today's procedure. He'll use the images from the CT scanner to guide the needle into my lung. I'll have local freezing and be awake for the entire procedure, since breathing at exactly the same rate and depth throughout the test is crucial.

He begins by taking a few images to locate the general area of the mass. After administering the freezing, he punctures my right side with a large bore needle. I wince despite the freezing. When the table automatically moves inside the scanner, I lie with the needle dangling from my side, breathing as instructed. The doctor returns to the small booth, takes a number of images, and returns to advance the needle further into my side. The pain is excruciating because the needle is beyond the frozen layer of flesh. He keeps repeating the same steps. The procedure, painful and meticulous, is taking forever. Maintaining the breathing pattern is becoming almost impossible.

The needle has to be into the lung. "No," he announces, "we're not inside the lung yet." The pain is incapacitating, now. What is it going to be like when he finally enters the lung? Small tears form at the outside corners of my eyes. The stress and pain are starting to take their toll. I'm not as brave as I care to think. I prepare for the pain to come. My chest aches, and each breath reminds me of the object piercing my flesh.

"I'm ready to perforate the lung," he warns.

I've braced myself, but it's not enough. The final advance is indescribable. My chest is paralyzed. The table moves back into the scanner for final images. Summoning all my resolve doesn't alleviate my predicament. I think of my pediatric babies with chest tubes. What endless suffering they had to endure.

The table slides out of the scanner. The needle has managed to pierce the mass. Standing at my right side ready to obtain the biopsy specimen, the doctor inserts the biopsy gun through the tunnel of the large bore needle. Pressure builds inside my lung. The gun clicks when he gathers the first of three specimens.

The wave of sickness is unexpected and takes a bizarre twist. Dizzy and tingling, I feel the urgency to cough rise from deep within my lung. There's something in my throat.

"I have to cough," I cry out.

"Stay still, we're almost finished," he commands.

Tears continue to slip silently down my cheeks. I've reached my limit. The sensation to cough is overwhelming.

The dressing stretches across my side, a temporary seal while my lung heals. I can cough. I cover my mouth with my hands. My first cough is painful, yet relieves the sensation in my lung. My hands are covered in blood! The doctor notices the expression of horror on my face and informs me that expectorating blood for the first few hours is normal.

I lie on the stretcher in the hall waiting for a chest x-ray, clutching the bleach-white hospital towel, the dark red blood making a bold statement to those who pass. No one has taken my vital signs to evaluate my recovery, yet the area is bustling with people.

The x-ray technician tells me I must me sit up.

"No," I retort, "I'm in too much pain. If you want x-rays, you'll have to take them with me lying down." I'm in no mood to comply with ridiculous requests.

Back into the hall, I bide my time for another thirty minutes before a porter can transport me back to my room. No one has checked on me. If no one is interested in taking my vital signs, I'll have to take my own.

Mom is calmly waiting in my room. A true stoic, she rarely reveals her real emotions, during times of stress. For the first time since I have been sick, a look of fear flashes across her face when she sees the bloody towel and my pale face. The glimpse into her mind is fleeting. Immediately, she composes herself, smiles, and greets me with her usual voice. I wonder how she does it, but I'm glad she can. Her strength is contagious and it helps to diminish my fear.

An experienced and competent nurse is attending me. I can tell that I'm in good hands by her mannerisms and the way in which she assesses me.

The pain is more bearable and my appetite has returned. It's difficult to eat lying on my right side, so Mom is assisting me. I glance over at the blood pressure gauge, which is recording every fifteen minutes. 85/40, very low! I gulp down three large cups of water, hoping to correct the situation. I can't let my blood pressure fall any lower.

Having Mom here makes the time pass quickly. We laugh and make light of whatever we can. I had always tried to make the situation humorous, when appropriate, for my cancer patients. I'm beginning to realize the importance of that philosophy to healing, physically and spiritually.

GOOD NEWS!! The biopsy sample doesn't show any evidence of cancer. Mom and I laugh and hug each other. I'm not going to die.

Doctor ID1 suspects a fungal infection in my lung. However, it will take several weeks for the lab to culture and identify the mass, and he'll have to wait for culture results to make a definite diagnosis. Medication will also have to wait until after the preliminary biopsy report, which will be available in a few days. We discuss the lung test results. They indicate that my lungs are diffusing sufficient oxygen to the tissues, but I'm hyperventilating. He suggests that breathing into a paper bag will alleviate the shortness of breath. With that remark, he leaves.

I'm furious and insulted. Hyperventilation is not a problem during my nocturnal attacks. I've timed the respirations myself, always normal at twenty-four per minute. Of course I was hyperventilating the morning of the test. I breathed faster because I was scared, sick, and felt as if my throat was closing. Everybody appears so casual about my problem. Is this all about making money? More tests and more money. Is that the name of the game. What about me?

The nurse enters my room and hands me a paper bag. Doctor ID1 has actually written an order for a paper bag! To make fun of the situation, I cut two holes for eyes, place the bag over my head, and put my glasses over top of the bag. Mom and I laugh at this ridiculous situation while she takes my picture. The bag quickly finds its way into the garbage.

The eight o'clock announcement signals the end of visiting hours and Mom's departure. I don't look forward to the night with its dreaded episodes. But my side is feeling better. A pain killer is suppressing the lingering discomfort from the biopsy, an annoyance which now floats off in the distance. What a great discovery! I'll take a pain killer to help me deal with my symptoms.

## October 8

What a refreshing change to awaken to the sound of a breakfast tray. I'm feeling better than I have in days.

However, the day drags by with the usual parade of doctors coming to see me. Discussing our plans for the evening, Mom and I anticipate spending time together—somewhere other than in my hospital room—as we wait for Doctor ID1 to discharge me. We're ready to go home.

The student nurse, making her early evening assessments, notices that the left side of my mouth is drooping and asks how I'm feeling. I reply that the left side of my face is numb. She checks my pupils and finds that the left one is slightly dilated and responding sluggishly to the light test. As we discuss this, I my eyes are burning, the left side of my neck is red, and the tingling and numbness have returned to my left arm.

By the time Doctor N1 arrives on rounds, the numbness has subsided, and my facial functions have returned to normal. After examining me, he dismisses the nurse's concerns as invalid. He doesn't believe the numbness and tingling are physical symptoms, a conclusion he substantiates with evidence from the MRI scan which revealed no abnormalities. Normal. Everything appears normal except my lung.

Doctor ID1 has finally arrived. No preliminary biopsy results as yet, but he'll discharge me. I'm to contact him next week. We discuss my trip to Paris. He vetoes any travel that will take me away from my specialized care, and Mom agrees with his decision. Deep down, I know they're both right. I turn my head to hide my disappointment.

I don't feel comfortable leaving without a detailed plan for treatment, but Mom has to leave for Canada in the morning, and I want to spend my last night with her at home. Happily, I shed my hospital gown, faint signs of trouble gnawing at the edges of my consciousness as I dress. Must be the excitement of going home, butterflies. Mom has loaded the truck and parked it in front of the hospital entrance. I know when I climb out of the wheelchair and into the truck that my imagination is not playing tricks on me. I'm ill. The nausea comes in waves, and I retch for the entire drive home.

I collapse on the couch in my apartment. My face is burning; my abdomen, arms, and legs are on fire; and my ears are ringing. It's only 8 p.m. Already I feel worse than during most of my hospital stay.

I try to stand, but I can't. I cry out, "Mom, help me!"

"Heather, you should go back to the hospital. I'm going to call." Mom phones the hospital.

"They say you can't return without a doctor's order for readmission. What do you want me to do? I can't leave you alone tomorrow morning when you're sick."

This is supposed to be our special night together, instead our stress levels mount with the onslaught of each symptom. Mom's flight is early in the morning. She's afraid to leave me, and I'm afraid to be by myself. We have arranged for Don's Mom to take care of me for the next two weeks. Jean isn't scheduled to arrive for a few days.

For the first time Mom breaks down in front of me. I don't want to make her cry or feel guilty for leaving. She doesn't want to leave, but she must return to work. I'm supposed to be better, instead I'm worse. As I watch Mom's tears fall, I know I have to summon more courage. I can't let her know how scared I really am. Somehow, I have to find the strength to manage. After a few chaotic minutes, we dry our tears. Time to devise a practical, interim solution. I decide to call Onnie, who has offered to help me, if I need anything. Although I don't know her very well, I have to impose, to surrender my independence. I can see the relief on Mom's face once Onnie has agreed and the arrangements are finalized.

As the symptoms bombard my body, Mom bathes me. The warm bath brings temporary relief. I take a pain killer to suppress the symptoms, and falling into bed, hope to escape through sleep.

**October 9**

The symptoms have returned with renewed vigor and prod me awake. I take more pain killers. "Sleep. Just let me sleep."

I know by her movements that Mom is awake beside me. The chills and shaking are beginning, and she reaches over to hold me, trying to alleviate my fear with compassion.

Even though I haven't slept since the last attack, the comfort of Mom's arms has given me the security to brave the night. As the time for her departure approaches, I know she senses my panic.

Mom hugs me good-bye, and I put on a brave face. Both of us are aware of my terror, but we must choose to ignore it. The door closes. I cry. I take more pain killers. My tears eventually cease, and I slip into sleep.

The phone is ringing. No, the ringing is in my ears. Walking toward the bathroom, I lose my balance and fall. I'm having trouble standing upright. Waves of nausea engulf me, as the numbness creeps into my left side. Knowing I have to eat to keep up my strength, I stumble to the fridge, eat a few bites of chicken before tumbling back into bed.

Onnie has arrived. I thank her for coming and explain that I'm unable to be sociable. This is unusual for me. I am by nature a very social person, always happy and enthusiastic. Today will have to be an exception. I hurt all over. Onnie understands.

## The Toxic Labyrinth

I can hear noise, constant static invading the luxury of my sleep. Someone has left the TV on when the station is off the air. The sound echoes though my head, louder and louder. I push my mind into consciousness. Where's the TV? The sound doesn't go away. It's inside my head. My face, my eyes, the inside of my nose are burning. My head is screaming in pain, and my entire left side is numb. I try to force my hand to close, but it won't comply.

"Onnie," I call out in desperation, "I have to go back to the hospital."

The same room. The all too familiar staff. I watch the IV solution drip into my wrist. I'll have to phone Don in Africa. He expects me to be at home, and he'll worry if he calls and there's no answer. I must phone Jean. She's flying to Memphis in a few days. But I'll worry about these things tomorrow. I'm too tired tonight.

### October 10

A distant nagging wakes me. Numbness in my left arm has interrupted my peaceful sleep. My watch glows 3 a.m. Yes, my symptoms are right on schedule. I make a mental note of my discomfort and go back to sleep.

I awake refreshed, yet each muscle is stiff as if I have just completed a long marathon. Even though I'm feeling considerably better, I'm still unable to hold up my head. Sleep overtakes me once more, and I finally open my eyes at four in the afternoon. Why have I come back to the hospital? I feel so much better. What happens to make me so ill, only to vanish twelve hours later? However, these thoughts are short lived, and by evening, my symptoms have returned.

### October 12

Tests and more tests. The old routine has started again. My biopsy results indicate fungus as the most likely cause of the mass in my lung. Before Doctor ID1 will prescribe medicine, a spinal tap will be added to my growing list of unforgettable tests. Does my spinal fluid contain fungus? A large needle puncture into my spine will answer this question.

Thinking about the complications of paralysis and infection that can result from a lumbar puncture doesn't ease my mind. Some of my children had not functioned normally after this procedure due to these complications. My children on the cancer ward had lumbar punctures performed, as often as, every week. I had to hold their small bodies while the doctors administered freezing into the back and inserted the needle into the spine. The procedure made my skin crawl. Today my heart is heavy for those children for I can comprehend more easily the range of emotions they must have experienced. As a caregiver I could be sympathetic, but I could never truly empathize with their pain and suffering. Now that it's happening to me, I'm learning first hand the reality of chronic illness.

With each passing minute my apprehension grows. The knock on the door shatters the silence of my sanctuary. Doctor N1 has arrived.

"Have you eaten dinner?" I inquire.

"Yes," he answers.

I breathe a sigh of relief. He won't hurry with the procedure: a steady hand is important.

Instruments thud on a steel tray. Bent over at the waist, my head between my knees, my legs hanging over the edge of the bed, I grip the stuffed animal I'm holding even tighter.

"Ready?" he asks.

I close my eyes and mutter a little prayer, "Please don't miss." I had watched many doctors poke the spinal needle into a child and proceed to dig around aimlessly looking for the right spot. The child would writhe and cry, which made the process all the more tortuous to watch. Sometimes it would have to be redone. If the child was old enough to understand, I would give the hand I was holding a reassuring squeeze. I always wondered if that gesture had made any difference. Right now I wish someone would give my hand a reassuring squeeze.

The first needle pierces my flesh. The freezing fluid burns slightly, then intensifies as more of the medication flows under my skin, the liquid creating pressure when it separates the tissue in my back. I clench my jaw. Each minute is an hour. More jabs. More freezing. The shaft of the needle sinks into my back up to the hub, producing an abrupt and lingering pain. I suck in my breath as the burning increases. The third needle is not so invasive. The freezing in my back is starting to take effect.

"Dear God, don't let me feel anything," I plead silently.

I can visualize the large and unusually long needle. Doctor N1 warns me to indicate immediately if my extremities go numb, eradicating the confidence that I've summoned to this point. I push the thought about paralysis to the back of my mind and divert my thoughts by counting one, two, three . . .

The band-aid is in place, a temporary seal for my back while the puncture heals. If I have to lie flat, how will I avoid going to the bathroom for the next six hours? I would rather die than ask for the bedpan.

Jean has arrived! She'll help take my mind off things. The situation is rather ironic. Jean has traveled all the way to Memphis to nurse a virtual stranger. What a way to get acquainted with my future mother-in-law, to develop a friendship within the confines of my hospital room. While I regain my health, we'll be roommates for the next few weeks, a closeness that should make or break our relationship.

Regardless of what is happening in my life, it's important for me to entertain a guest. I suspend thoughts about my health and put on my best behavior to impress my future mother-in-law. It's show time!

The time of the day that I dread most is approaching. I miss Mom. I miss Don. How do I confide my fears to Jean? Will having her stay with me be stressful? Everyday is stressful for me right now.

Since I've always been independent, I resent this sudden change. I'm uncomfortable relying on someone else, especially someone I barely know. Jean is here to pacify Don. I'll be able to manage on my own in about a week and have no intention of playing the invalid.

A nurse peeks her head into the room and inquires whether I need to use the bedpan. I decide to assert my independence and shake my head, no. During the next two hours, I may regret my decision, but I try not to concentrate on my already full bladder. No giving in, I can wait. The nurse leaves without assessing me. I wonder what she'll document on my chart. Because she did not examine me, I decide to do this myself. I reach around to my back and touch the band-aid site. It's still dry and intact. No spinal fluid has leaked out.

**October 13**

It's almost 1:30 a.m. My chest tightness is right on schedule, but subsides quickly, allowing me concentrate on the TV. Now that my disease has a cause, my situation is a little less scary. The symptoms haven't changed, but dealing with a specific disease is less intimidating. I'm not as afraid as I was now that I have a cause to focus on, to fight against.

Another day dawns and another test looms on the horizon. The bone marrow aspirate will determine whether the fungal infection has spread to my bone marrow.

The nurse injects a sedative while the lab assistant sets up the slides on the table beside my bed. A young doctor enters. My nurse has assured me of his competence. The nurse will always confirm, if the doctor is good, and will make no comment, if there is something to worry about.

The doctor's bedside manner puts me immediately at ease, and I roll onto my side exposing my hip. The first freezing needle penetrates. Exerting more force on the second needle, he drives it deeper, burying the shaft against the bone. I grit my teeth while he repeats this procedure three more times.

## The Toxic Labyrinth

Finally, it's time to apply the large bore needle and remove the bone marrow. The doctor puts his weight behind the twisting motion, rotating the needle towards the bone. He stops. More freezing is required. My body language indicates I can feel the needle. Three more stabs of freezing fluid. Another attempt to puncture the bone, but I can still feel the needle. He explains that younger people tend to have more sensitive coverings on the bone. Is this statement supposed to reassure me?

He resumes the twisting motion, causing surges of pain. Tears stream silently down my face, and I grab the bed rail for support. The crunching of the bone when he gathers each sample seems to fill the room. He warns me that the last sample will be even more painful, because he has to break off a small fragment of the bone for the lab.

Jean sits in the chair beside my bed. I can't hide my tears. The whole experience has been traumatic. I place my independence on hold, knowing I need Jean's help to get through this. I'm worn out; I'm not the same strong, fearless person I was two weeks ago. Jean comforts me with her wisdom and soft words of support, intuitively knowing how to expel my fear. I'm glad she's here.

The sedative that the nurse injected at the beginning of the procedure is finally starting to work. It was supposed to be effective during the procedure, not now. My tears withdraw further and further into the distance. The room is warm and safe. I sleep.

I force myself awake through the fogginess of the sedative. No one has checked my dressing! Maybe I'm bleeding.

I call to Jean, "Is there any blood on the dressing?" She assures me there is none. No blood. The words echo in my mind as the remaining effects of the sedative seduce my body into slumber.

**CHAPTER 3**

# MIRAGE

Off in the distance the illusion shimmers, enticing me toward
the safety of its shores.

# The Toxic Labyrinth

## October 14

Time to leave the hospital! I'm anxious to erase the events of the past three weeks from my mind, as quickly as possible. Armed with a diagnosis and medication, I'm confident that rest in familiar surroundings is the ticket to recovery. Feeling more energetic than the last time I was discharged, I pack slowly without having to fight waves of nausea.

The walk from the parking lot to the pharmacy is half a city block, but to my sluggish body it appears to be a mile. Three hundred and fifty dollars for three weeks of medicine, and the clerk won't accept a personal check. I turn to look out the window of the pharmacy. From down the block, the brightly lit logo on the bank machine sends a message—cash, cash. I have no choice, but to make the effort. A mental picture of home and my inviting bed spurs me on.

## October 15 to October 27

Sleep and rest, rest and sleep. For the first few days, I could stay awake for only two hours before sleep would entice my body. I had taken a few weeks leave from work, and with Jean handling all the household chores, I could focus on my recovery.

I wanted to act as tour guide and show Jean the sights and sounds of Memphis, but I had to save my strength for our short outings on the weekends. No matter what I wanted, my body was dictating my routine.

Although the joint pains were diminishing, I was still dealing with arthritic-like pains. Each day I would limber up my joints before getting out of bed. Walking was often painful in the morning, because my back and hips ached so much. At times the discomfort in my hands made holding a book, cutting with scissors, or opening a jar lid arduous. My difficulties made it easy for me to relate to the elderly who are plagued with these problems daily.

As the days progressed, my strength gradually returned, the symptoms became less intense, my waking hours expanded, and the interrupted nights were only an occasional annoyance. The frozen hands, burning nerves, crushing chest pain, and shaking episodes were becoming a distant memory.

Jean had to leave before Don returned from Nigeria. Having her with me for the recovery period, had been a blessing. For the two nights before Don arrived, I was nervous being alone, but the time passed without incident. It had been a long month since Don's departure in September. So much had happened. It was hard to believe all my hospital adventures had occurred during his absence.

I felt better than I had in a long time. Although the recurring pain in my left hand and periodic numbness on my left side bothered me during the day, I was certain these remaining symptoms would disappear once the medication destroyed the fungus.

**October 28 to November 11**

Don will walk off the plane in a few minutes. I watch for his tall frame. There he is! The familiar sauntering gait and blond curly mane bring tears of joy. He gathers me in his arms, and all is well with my world.

We're disappointed that our trip to Paris had to be canceled. As we discuss the events of the last month, Don reveals his secret plan. He had made arrangements to propose to me in Paris. Sadness wells up inside, as I think about my special surprise.

"When you are better, we will take that trip to Paris," Don assures me. "Getting better is the most important plan for you at the moment."

## The Toxic Labyrinth

Instead of Paris, he has planned a ten day trip to Houston, Galveston, and New Orleans. While Don attends business seminars, I will enjoy the sights and rest. Will I feel well enough to go?

The day of the trip has arrived. Don is taking charge of all the packing, so I can rest. I'm excited. I feel fine.

As the plane leaves the runway, I'm surprised by the sudden recurrence of tightness in my chest, the feeling of claustrophobia and suffocation. Everything is closing in around me. I can't breathe. An asthma attack. I reach for my inhaler. A couple of puffs produce immediate relief.

Being away from Memphis and my doctors for a number of days makes me apprehensive. Don must have interpreted my thoughts. He reaches over to hold my hand, giving it an affectionate squeeze. I snuggle against him, gaining strength from this solid, dependable man.

Houston is a tonic for my health. During the day I rest and in the evening I accompany Don to business dinners. I still experience the occasional night of interrupted sleep when numbness on my left side nudges me awake, and my joints are stiff intermittently, with the exception of my left wrist, which seems to hurt all the time. A hot bath eases most of my discomforts, so I'm spending more and more time in the tub.

In Galveston, a quaint city on the gulf, our charming room in a Victorian bed and breakfast awaits us. Dining by the ocean, we talk about rescheduling our Paris trip. Later, as we stroll through the turn of the century neighborhoods, holding hands, we plan our future by spinning dreams about a home, children, and our career paths.

On the surface I appear happy, but in the back of my mind nagging doubts remain. I continue to experience periods of sickness which frighten me. Occasionally, I wake in the night feeling unwell. Don holds me, brushing away my tears and fearfulness. With him at my side, I feel a little braver.

Doctor ID1 told me I would have to take the medication for at least a year to eliminate the fungus. The symptoms won't disappear immediately. I will have to be patient, a trait I'll have to develop.

We've arrived in New Orleans, our special city where Don and I discovered love amid the pleasures of jazz, the French Quarter, Cajun dancing, and fine dining. We both have wonderful memories of the city. I had to cancel a trip to New Orleans my first weekend in the hospital. Now, I can make up for that loss.

I'm more energetic in New Orleans than I was in Houston and Galveston. Don and I explore the sights, visit friends, and dance to Cajun music at one of our favorite haunts. Am I finally turning the corner?

**November 13 to November 16**

Our first trip since the onset of my illness was so successful we have decided to be adventurous, and have planned a short tour through western Tennessee before Don's return to Nigeria.

Two large dogs lie on the floor of the smoky hotel office, the only lodging of choice in this small town. The woman behind the desk is very chatty and wants to talk. Cigarette smoke hangs in the air, the haze enveloping us as we stand listening politely to her conversation. Finally, I tug impatiently at Don's sleeve until he understands that I have to lie down.

I lean on Don all the way back to the room. Tired of feeling ill, I lie on the bed and start to cry. "Don, I'm afraid I may never get well. Suppose I die. Will you miss me?"

"Don't say such things. Of course I'll miss you. I would be very lonely without you."

Don hugs me and encourages me to be strong.

"Don, I'll always love you. If something happens to me, I'll never truly be gone. I'll watch over you every day. I'll be beside you in spirit and lie with you every night. You'll feel my presence and know that I'm there. You'll never be without me."

He buries his head in my hair. "Stop saying those things. You're going to get better." He holds me for a very long time, while he wipes away my tears.

Quaint Bell Buckle, our destination. Nestled in a postcard-like setting, the local bed and breakfast, a most inviting mansion, becomes home for a few days. French doors open into our room, which is furnished with antiques and decorated in country elegance. It's not Paris, but the setting is just as romantic. The location doesn't matter as long as we are together. Leaving our worries behind, we explore the Tennessee countryside, have fun, and laugh.

**November 17**

Doctor ID1 asks how I'm feeling, and I mention the intermittent numbness on my left side. He explains that the fungus could be causing the numbness, but the problem should eventually disappear. The rest of me checks out fine.

**November 18**

I've started to wake up every third night with chills. The clock always indicates an identical pattern with my previous symptoms, between two and three in the morning. What's the meaning of this pattern? Why do my symptoms assert themselves at the same time every night?

Don helps me through each incident and brings me what I crave, usually a piece of bread, to clear the nausea. He holds me until I fall back to sleep. He knows the spells scare me and that I don't like to be awake and alone while they last. But Don's time with me is drawing to an end. What will I do if these night sessions continue?

# Mirage

**November 19**

I lie down and turn out the light. Bright colors dance across the dark room. Are the colors from looking into the light before I turned it off? I turn on the light. The colors remain, pulsating colors of green, gold, red, blue, and pink which resemble a stained glass window. I cover my left eye, vision normal. I cover my right eye and watch the colors continue their wild dance, while the vision in my left eye quickly fades.

"Don, I can't see!"

We're both afraid. What should we do? We decide to remain calm. Will the next few minutes give us some direction? Don brings me a piece of bread, as he has each time I have my spells during the night. How will eating a piece of bread restore my vision? We don't know. It's all we can think of. Fearfully we hold on to each other willing my vision to return.

Twenty minutes has elapsed. The silvery blindness is receding and my vision is returning in stages. An intense headache, which spreads across both eyes and down into the base of my neck, serves to remind me of this bizarre incident. We'll notify Doctor ID1 first thing in the morning.

Doctor ID1 hasn't returned my call. However, I appear to be back to normal, except for the annoying headache.

Don and I are determined to enjoy our last few days together, before he returns to Africa. We walk in the park, crushing the multicolored, autumn leaves beneath our feet. We run through the woods chasing each other, reveling in the power of our love for one another.

Our day in the woods has been invigorating. The musty smell of the leaves hasn't made my chest tight. Recalling our trip to England and Wales last March, I remember my intolerance for the smell of mold or damp musty places. The old buildings made my chest tight, and we had to be choosy about our lodgings, quite a feat since most places are old and dank. Now I can tolerate the damp autumn woods. Is this a good omen?

Our last evening together in Memphis calls for a special treat. One of our favorite diversions is dining in upscale, trendy restaurants. We always plan our own restaurant tour when we move to a new city, and Memphis is no exception.

Gazing into Don's eyes, I think how lucky I am to have this special man in my life. We've dressed more formally for this occasion, and he looks especially handsome. We discuss wedding arrangements, deciding that next summer or fall would give me enough time to plan. As far as Don is concerned, we could get married tomorrow, although he does want a romantic setting to propose formally. He'll make arrangements for our Paris trip as soon as I'm well enough to travel that far. He's revised his plans, ones that will remain secret until the time is right. How can I help but love this man? He's such a romantic.

The menu at Paulette's displays the inventiveness of the chef. The fresh salmon reminds me of my home on the west coast. We always have wine on these special occasions. I forego the alcohol settling for an after dinner cappuccino instead. My health is important. I'll be drinking wine soon enough.

I awaken from my sleep with a start. There's no pain, only agitation and restlessness. Don rolls over and presses me against his body. Twenty minutes pass before I start to shake. Don holds me tighter, trying to dissolve the tremors. The jittery feeling disappears with the shaking, leaving me exhausted. As my eyes become heavy and begin to close, Don whispers that he loves me. With his reassuring words echoing in my mind, I drift off to sleep.

**November 22**

The phone rings insistently.

"Hello."

Doctor ID1's office is finally inquiring about my loss of vision. The receptionist is extremely anxious to make an appointment. Is she trying to cover for herself because my message didn't reach the doctor last Friday? The crisis was three days ago, and I see no need for an examination. Don convinces me that an appointment would be wise, and I agree to make the visit after I take him to the airport.

No matter how many times I say good-bye to Don, I always cry. Watching him walk up the ramp, knowing it will be another month until I see him again is the part of our life I'll never adjust to. I don't care if people stare. Crying, I hug him over and over again. He's always the brave one and reassures me that he will return. At a time like this, it's so hard to be in love. Every month a part of me goes with him. From the time I watch the airplane doors close, I start counting the hours until he returns.

Doctor ID1 wants me to return next Monday after I have seen Doctor N1 about losing my vision. Driving home from the doctor's office, I am determined to think pleasant thoughts rather than dwell on Don's departure. Christmas plans. He'll be home for Christmas, our first Christmas together. I'll decorate the apartment. Maybe I can work on my cooking skills and cook a turkey.

Restlessness and agitation hover in the background. The day has been stressful. That's probably the reason.

What do I do first, now that Don is gone? I hate cooking, but I hate it even more when Don is away. I used to come home from work, dreading the thought of preparing a meal. Always tired after my shift and a thirty minute commute, I usually boiled spaghetti, heated up something from a package, or grabbed dinner from the local fast food outlet. Recently, I've discovered frozen dinners, a great invention. What could be more suited to my time-constrained life style than this simple to open box with the little plastic compartmentalized tray that can be heated in the microwave. An entree from the freezer makes lunch an easy decision. A meal in an instant.

As I lie on the couch laughing at a funny scene on the evening sit com, waves of agitation ebb and flow, each wave increasing in intensity. By 11:00 p.m., the agitation becomes extreme, dominating my thoughts. A pain killer will suppress the symptoms.

The agitation has changed to a generalized tingling across my back and neck. Nausea makes me retch. The symptoms that I thought were gone are creeping back one by one. Now that I'm alone, I'm beginning to become concerned. My hands are frozen. Short of breath, I gasp for air. Severe chills penetrate my body, causing it to shake uncontrollably. I have to make it to the bathroom. The room is whirling. More nausea. I retch. I vomit.

"Keep calm. You have to pull through this. You're alone. It's up to you," I tell myself. The fungus must be back. That's what's making me so sick. Fortifying my courage, I tighten my grip on the edges of the toilet.

It's over. The sickness has stopped, as quickly as it started. The calm after the storm. All is well again.

The phone rings and it's Don calling from London. I tell him that the sickness seems to be back. Although I don't understand this monster that possesses me without warning, his comforting words calm me for the moment. My sister's voice comes on the line. Don is visiting with her on his stopover. Rhonda and I chat, but all too soon the conversation is over. I hang up the phone and begin to cry as the images of Don and Rhonda, so far away, crowd my mind.

**November 23**

Who would be phoning at 2 a.m.? Don is calling to make certain I'm all right. Our desultory conversation centers around his visit with Rhonda and her life in London. His voice sounds so far away. I miss him, but I have to be brave. In the background, I hear the boarding announcement for Don's flight to Nigeria and with this, he blows me a good-bye kiss, sending his love, and is gone.

The waves of nausea have wakened me. My shoulder blades are aching, and the palm of my left hand is burning. I lie awake, the unwilling prisoner of my symptoms. Every hour on the hour, the burning nerves and agitation have jolted me out of my sleep. Each thirty minute episode has culminated in tremors which have left me exhausted. I drift back to sleep, wondering how long the peace will last. I have started to scribble the times and symptoms down on a piece of paper. The time has come to keep detailed records.

I have awakened in the late morning feeling much improved. What can Doctor N1 do for me? I'm already on medication. Maybe he'll have some answers on Monday.

The day has passed with some intermittent periods of agitation and tingling, but nothing compared to the night before.

Another evening sprawled in front of the TV. My days revolve around this black box of Don's, because I have little energy for much else. Funny how my life has changed in such a short time. Until now, I had too many other activities to occupy my time and have never owned a TV. Out of touch with this medium, I found the pastime relaxing at first. Reruns of shows I remembered from my childhood were familiar, and the popular prime time shows and characters presented a new experience. After almost two months of this diversion, the novelty has worn off. Although I need the relaxation, it is no longer entertaining.

To make certain my attention is not fully occupied by the figures on the screen, I'm distracted by my constant companions—tingling in my face, burning in my left eye, ringing in my ears, numbness on the left side of my face, and throbbing on the left side of my neck.

# The Toxic Labyrinth

**November 25**

I have called Mom to talk about my progress.

"Heather, your worst symptoms seem to be around eight in the evening and three in the morning. There must be some reason why they appear around the same time every day. Why do you feel so much better in the morning? Are you doing something at the same time during the day to make yourself so ill? There must be some reason for this pattern. It's as if something you are eating is poisoning you."

"I don't know, Mom."

"Maybe you have an allergy to something you're eating. Are you eating something different that you weren't eating before?"

"No. Besides, I'm not eating at three in the morning when I have these episodes. I don't know why I should start feeling sick now that Don is gone."

I fall asleep with Mom's words tucked away in the back of my mind. Poisoned. That's exactly how I have been feeling lately. If I'm being poisoned, what could be the cause? Nothing in my life has changed.

**November 26**

Where am I? Who am I? I can't feel my hands. It's still dark. What does the clock say? 5:30. I'm in my bed in Memphis. I can't move my legs. I have to get up and walk, but I'm confused. How do I make my body work? My nerves are on fire. I have to move. I have to throw up. Help, I need help. My mind races while it functions in this confused and disoriented manner.

I have dragged myself to the kitchen to get a drink of water, but I can't hold on to the glass. I have to try again. I look at the faucet, wondering how it works. After what seems like an eternity, I remember how to turn it on, and force myself to drink the glass of water. Thankfully, I still know how to drink

Something is dreadfully wrong. Someone has to help me.

Daryl, my friend Daryl. It's so hard to think. I pick up the phone and stare at it. I can't remember how to dial. I have to concentrate, because I know how to do this. Slowly my mind starts to clear. The shaking, the most violent I've ever experienced, makes my teeth chatter.

Finally, it's over, and the frozen feeling leaves my hands. I lie awake. The pounding of my heart accentuates my fear. Previous episodes of confusion have never lasted as long or been as debilitating. I have to call Doctor N1 today. I can't wait until Monday. Why am I becoming more and more nauseated as the days pass? I doze for short periods, but nausea or pain keep interrupting my peace.

Eight in the morning on the Thanksgiving long weekend, and the doctor-on-call is the only one available. Once again I relate my long history and explain last night's incident. Although I'm having trouble concentrating, I have to find the words to convey my concern. The doctor is no help, and states that I should wait to be tested by Doctor N1 on Monday. But Monday is so far away. What do I do next? My health doesn't appear to be improving. I have to devise a plan.

I'm certain Daryl will help me. He visited me in the hospital and is familiar with my problem. When I phone and describe my latest symptoms, he agrees to stay with me during the night.

I've planned a trip home to Canada for ten days, leaving December 2nd. Can I hang on until I get there? I'm fearful of leaving my doctors in Memphis. They know my complex history and are the only people who can help me. My condition is too complicated, beyond any experience I've encountered as a nurse. The doctors in Canada rarely encounter a fungal infection, except in cancer patients who have been on potent drugs to suppress their immune systems.

# The Toxic Labyrinth

Doctor ID1 thinks I've been exposed to a fungus that's native to the southwestern US desert. What do Canadian doctors know about such a condition? But I want to go home, to be with Mom for a few days, to gain reassurance.

I have called my girlfriend, Grace, who is a physician. She knows about my condition and reassures me that the doctors in Memphis are very competent and are giving me good care.

I know that fungus takes a long time to cure. My children suffering from cancer who also had fungus took a very long time to recover, and in fact, some never did. That last thought sticks in my mind. Many of my children didn't recover. Will that be my fate? Is the fungus residing in my brain and causing my periods of confusion? I have to stop thinking these thoughts. Negative thinking won't make me well. With this, a wave of nausea washes over me. Is the fungus winning? I have to be strong enough to fly home.

## November 27

Daryl is staying with me at night, and although I'm not feeling any better, having someone in the other room gives me the strength to endure the night.

I'm sick all the time. Shortness of breath. Nausea. Ringing in my ears. Aching joints. Shaking. Retching. Nerves on fire. Sometimes I lose the grip in my hands. I have difficulty walking. My symptoms have always been the worst at night. Now I'm beginning to feel sick in the mornings as well. Monday can't come too quickly.

## November 28

I have planned a small surprise engagement party for my friend, Cindy. Even though Daryl has tried to dissuade me, I'm pushing myself, believing that preparations for the party will take my mind off my problems.

Cindy wants the whole world to celebrate with her on the day she becomes engaged. She loves hockey, so her boyfriend has planned to surprise her. He will ask for her hand in front of all the fans, after the first period of the Memphis Kings' hockey game. He has cut a hockey puck in half, hinged it, lined it with velvet, and placed the ring inside. I want to see the look on her face.

I hurriedly finish a frozen dinner and jump into the car. The pressure intensifies in my chest as I drive, and my hands can't feel the steering wheel. The road markings are swimming in front of my eyes. The nausea rises from the pit of my stomach, and I have to pull over. Why can I never predict when I'm going to get sick? I want to go to the game, but I can't hold my head up. I'll be lucky if I can drive home.

The party swirls around me, the couch potato hostess. Daryl has pitched in to help, leaving me free to entertain my guests without expending much energy or aggravating my condition. Despite my disappointment at missing the actual engagement, I am pleased by the success of the party.

**November 29**

Doctor N1 will have some suggestions because he'll know why my symptoms are getting worse. Appearing to concentrate intently on what I have to say, he listens as I explain my temporary loss of vision and the escalation of my other symptoms. When I finish, he inquires about the cancellation of my marriage plans and the trip to Paris. What, if anything, does that have to do with my loss of vision and numbness in my arm?

"Your loss of vision is due to migraine headaches."

"Migraine headaches!" I argue with him. "How can one incident of vision loss be explained as migraine headaches? I never have headaches."

# The Toxic Labyrinth

As he scribbles a prescription for an anti-depressant, he explains that my other symptoms are the result of panic attacks and anxiety. I stare at him in disbelief. I waited until Monday for these ridiculous suggestions! Angrily, I push myself off the examining table, fling open the door, and look him straight in the eye.

"Can you tell me what relation a one inch mass in the chest and large red spots on the lower extremities have to anxiety?"

He weakly replies that those particular conditions are not his specialties. What kind of answer is this? I punctuate his last remark by slamming the door on my way out.

Furious, I storm out to the car. I had spent the whole weekend thinking I was going to die, only to be diagnosed as anxious. I have an appointment with Doctor ID1 this afternoon. He'll listen to me.

Still steaming when I arrive at Doctor ID1's office, I begin to experience waves of nausea which make it difficult for me to sit up. He asks me what Doctor N1 had to say, and I tell him, knowing that they'll eventually discuss the diagnosis. I also relate what has happened over the past week. Doctor ID1 indicates that I could have too much fungal medication in my system, which may account for my nausea, and recommends that I stop taking the medication for a while. However, the other symptoms are definitely not related to the fungal infection. How can this be? My symptoms haven't changed. I'm experiencing the same symptoms as I had in the hospital. During my last visit, he had told me that the numbness was due to neuropathy caused by the fungus. I pointedly ask what he intends to do. He's the kind of man that doesn't like to be confronted, but I'm mad and don't care. Answering cautiously, he says that he'll wait for three more weeks and repeat the CT scan of my lung to see if the lesion has calcified. If it has, the medicine is working. The only other recourse would be surgery on my lung.

"Lung surgery? If this is all in my head, why would I need lung surgery?"

He tries to skirt the issue, but I repeat my question. Finally, he admits that he is not certain what is in my lung, since the lab was unable to culture a fungus from the biopsy. He can't pinpoint the cause of my symptoms.

"Am I well enough to travel?"

"Yes."

"Will you write me a note saying I'm well enough to travel?" If I should require hospitalization in Canada, I want the note for the insurance company.

"No."

I sense he's in agreement with his colleague that I'm a hysterical female, one who would benefit from an antidepressant. He mentions, again, the benefit of a paper bag if I start to hyperventilate. I'm furious when I leave his office, after receiving no support from my doctor for the second time in one day.

Mom and I have talked at least twice a day on the phone since Don left. Sometimes I have disturbed her very late at night when I am alone and afraid of the power of these episodes that awaken me. Tonight I spill out my anger over the day's events.

"Mom, I have to come home. The doctors there know me. They'll believe that I am ill, that my symptoms are real. They know I don't have time to play games. Why is this happening now when I'm the happiest I've ever been."

"Heather, until now we thought it was best for you to stay in Memphis. If these symptoms are not related to the mass in your lung, you have to come home. It's too hard for you to stay there with no one to take care of you."

**November 30**

It seems an eternity before I can leave for home. Nothing is simple. I have a coupon, but in order to use it, I have to fly out of Little Rock,

71

## The Toxic Labyrinth

Arkansas. Since I can no longer trust myself to drive, Daryl will take me there.

The nausea no longer comes in waves; it's continuous. I'm retching more often, the ringing in my ears is continuous, my nerves burn, and I'm shaking most of the time.

What should I be packing? I place one item in the suitcase, lie down for fifteen minutes, then struggle up to pack another. If such a simple task is taking the whole day, how will I manage the seven hour flight?

# CHAPTER 4

## FALSE HOPES

The Siren seduces me with soft comforting words, a clever enchantress who gives me only false hopes.

# The Toxic Labyrinth

## December 2

A knock on the door. Daryl has arrived to drive me to the airport in Little Rock. After answering the door, I return to the bedroom and collapse on the bed.

Daryl looks at me. "You need to go to the hospital, not the airport."

"No, the only place I want to go is home. I'm getting on that plane even if I die doing it." I take one final look around my apartment, intuitively knowing I won't return.

Daryl hands me some anti-nausea medicine and instructs me to take it. I know he's right, that I won't be able to endure the flight without drugging myself. Bread and milk are the only foods my stomach will accept. If I eat when Daryl is with me, he can pull over and help me if get ill. I don't dare eat during the flight. My stomach has to be empty in case I have bouts of nausea. There is no way I want to throw up in front of the other passengers. I take the anti-nausea medication and wash it down with milk.

I'm having trouble concentrating on the conversation with Daryl, so I close my eyes. As the car speeds past the cotton fields, stripped of their white spheres, I occasionally peer at the scenery. Glances at the moving landscape only increase my nausea, and I quickly resume my resting position. The sedating effect of the anti-nausea medicine finally starts to work, and I welcome the temporary escape.

Assuming that I won't be able to walk the distance to change planes when I arrive in Houston, Daryl arranges for special transportation. Usually the activity in an airport lounge captures my attention. Today I curl up on a bench and sleep, waiting for the departure announcement.

It is time to board and I attempt the walk to the gate. After a few feet, I admit that I can't walk without assistance, and Daryl brings me a wheelchair.

I slump in my non-reclining seat at the back of the plane, the loud noise of the engines and the smell of the toilets adding to my nausea. Why do I feel claustrophobic the minute I enter an airplane? It seems as if there is never enough air. I take more medicine and prepare myself for the flight.

The porter and automated cart make changing planes for the final leg of my journey less formidable. Only five more hours to Seattle. I am determined to make it.

The chorus of coughing around me is a reminder that this is flu season. Pulling my coat collar over my face is the only defense I have against this new threat. I look at my watch every few minutes. Are the hands really moving or has time stopped? The waves of sickness are growing in intensity. Shifting in my seat, I look out the window and wonder if I can take more medicine. No, it's too soon. I want to retch, but suppress the urge. Seats, trays, and passengers seem to weave and churn. Thank God, my body has started to shake, signaling that this barrage of symptoms will soon be over. Twenty minutes later the sensation stops, leaving black patches to cloud my vision. I close my eyes and pray for sleep.

Twelve hours from Memphis to Seattle and the worst part of this trek is over. Dad's welcoming face stands out from the crowd in the terminal. My excitement at seeing him and making it this far is overshadowed by the urgency to lie down. The worried expression on his face reinforces the fact that I'm very ill. In the back of my mind, the thought grows that I won't be returning to Memphis in time for Christmas.

The hotel is inviting. My rather stringent diet during the day has reduced my symptoms and made me ravenous. I choke down the chicken sandwich and French fries, a fast food fix. The shaking and chills are starting again, but I'm almost home. I fall into a sick sleep.

# The Toxic Labyrinth

### December 3

All responsibility for my safe arrival in Vancouver has been transferred to Dad. I recline my seat and close my eyes. Three more hours by car and I'll be at Mom's.

All I can stomach is a dry, plain hamburger. I swallow the unappetizing contents of the plastic container, as we speed toward Vancouver in the December rain. The energy I have for casual conversation is quickly exhausted, sapped by the crushing tightness which has enveloped my chest. My legs tingle and are numb from the knees down.

It was seven years ago, and I had forgotten. After I was diagnosed with Crohn's disease, a numbness had plagued my left leg for months, a sensation that eventually disappeared. I hadn't given it another thought until now. Retching disturbs my thoughts, and I grab the hamburger container as a safety precaution. Only thirty minutes more.

The familiar streets of Vancouver descend toward the water. Lights from the ski lifts glimmer on the North Shore mountains. I'm home, and Memphis seems light years away.

Dad has brought me as far as Mom's apartment. Although they live in the same area, my parents have been divorced for a number of years. I look up the flight of stairs. Mom holds out her arm, knowing I can't make the climb by myself. Can make it as far as the bed?

Our conversation is brief. Mom has to teach an evening class and Doug is out. I tell her that I can manage as long as I don't have to get off this bed. She takes the cellular phone just in case.

I clutch the edges of the toilet, willing the room to stop spinning. Since I have eaten very little today, I wonder what I could possibly throw up. I'm too weak to stand. If I crawl on my hands and knees, I think I can make it to the bed. A crushing sensation grips my chest, making me gasp. Shock waves of pain immobilize my hips. Why do I feel like I'm being poisoned?

The tears make it difficult to concentrate on the number Mom has written on the paper. She has to come home and help me.

The minutes tick by slowly and with every breath there is pain. The room is cloaked in a white haze. Mom has returned and phoned my friend, Grace. Although we spoke on the phone when I was in Memphis about my medical care, it's been a year since we last met, and requesting medical assistance is not the way I had envisioned our first visit together. Because she has been a close friend for the last five years, she won't think the problem is all in my head.

Hearing footsteps on the stairs, I can barely lift my head in greeting. This is not the way I want my friends to see me, gagging and retching, unable to carry on a conversation. Grace softly voices her concern and quickly makes arrangements for me to see an internist

The internist, Dr. Il, listens intently and calmly asks me questions. Can I concentrate long enough to relate my complex history? The nurse holds me in a sitting position for the examination, because I'm too nauseated and weak to manage myself. Half way through we have to pause so I can throw up.

I'm shaking and cold. Mom brings several blankets from the warmer to cover me. There are no available beds in the wards, and I'm scheduled to spend the night in the emergency room. With a medical team just a shout away, I feel secure.

GOOD NEWS! The x-ray of my chest shows no visible mass in my lung. No mass means no lung surgery. But, if the mass has disappeared, what's making me so ill?

It's time for Mom to leave for the night. She unclasps the crystal from around her neck. "My energy is part of this crystal. Rhonda gave this charm to me exactly four years ago, when she left for London. It's kept me well and brought me luck. Maybe it can do the same for you."

# The Toxic Labyrinth

The nurse is beside my bed holding a syringe filled with fluid. Medication for nausea, Doctor I1's orders. I refuse. My previous experience has made me wary of taking medication in any other form except pills. The nurse voices her annoyance. "How are you going to swallow a pill when you're so nauseated?"

"I'll manage." It's very important for me to maintain control. With each passing day, I'm learning more about my body's responses to outside interference. My children often lost control once they were admitted to hospital. One day they were playing outside and the next they were prisoners of the hospital routine. Needles, tests, medicine. No escape. They always thought they had been bad and that hospitalization was the punishment.

The pill works quickly in my empty stomach, and the chaos of the emergency room starts to fade.

## December 4

The rattle of the breakfast tray doesn't entice me. I'm not as nauseated as the night before, but I'm not ready for food.

The hospital requires my emergency room cubicle for an incoming patient. From my hallway location, I watch the hospital awaken. Stretchers rumble by carrying patients, some voicing their suffering in strident tones. The doctors and nurses, encased in the glass control room, speak hurriedly about patients and diagnoses. The dietary staff stack meal trays into a rack positioned next to my head.

Off to my room in the ward. I'm ready for some solace, but solace will have to wait since no one has alerted the floor staff to my arrival. The two hour wait in the hall doesn't matter. Help is close at hand.

The neurologist, Doctor N2, apologizes that he has to conduct an initial examination in the hallway. The tap of the reflex hammer exhibits the sluggishness on my left side. Puzzled with this response, he repeats the test and the reaction is the same. This result doesn't surprise me. My left side has been the focal point for my symptoms from the beginning.

How different this room on the ward is from my rather palatial private one in Memphis. Each tiny space, not much larger than the dimensions of the bed, is demarcated by a washed-out blue curtain. Three elderly roommates in various stages of decline lie subdued, victims of time. How prophetic! Hadn't I been thinking about the elderly during my collapse in Memphis? Now I feel like one of them. At least these women can take comfort in the fact that their bodies have outlasted mine by sixty years.

A different nurse, another explanation of my problem. As I recount the historical details of my case once more, the though occurs to me that perhaps I should have this on tape.

Another CT scan of my head has been ordered, and I remain firm that no contrast dye be used. The technician reads my records and assures me that this dye is different. Closing my eyes, I hope for a better experience than the one I had in Memphis. I can taste the metal from the solution as the contrast infuses into my vein. A wave of nausea passes quickly. Just as I thought, the results indicate my head is normal.

I'm too weak to bathe myself. As Mom helps me into the shower, I glance at the railings lining the walls and the shower chair in the corner. Old people, these aids are for old people. I'm not that helpless. Mom holds onto my body, assisting my feeble legs to stand long enough for me to finish. It takes a monumental effort to raise my arms above my head and wash my hair.

Nancy chats about events at work. What do I have to offer in return other than stories about hospitals, past and present? We have been friends since university, part of a quintet. Heather, Nancy, Jane, Val, and Jessie, friends who shared the growing pains of higher learning and residence life. I want to visit, to take part in the conversation with Nancy and Dad, but the crushing sensation in my upper body torments me. No matter how I position myself, I can't get comfortable. It's difficult to carry on a conversation and be sociable when my mind is occupied elsewhere.

## December 5

Slowly, I navigate the hall unaided. As I pass each doorway, confused, elderly patients beseech me for help. The constant moaning and crying rings in my ears. Is my future written in these pathetic faces?

Back in my room, I shake off these disturbing images. I'm improving, a good sign. Besides, a long hospital stay will be costly while I'm covered by American health insurance.

The results of today's pulmonary function test have indicated mild asthma that is alleviated by the use of an inhaler. My shortness of breath is obviously not an illusion.

## December 6

This afternoon the respiratory technician gave me a mask of salt water. I breathed the salty solution through the mask to give her a sample for analysis. The smell of the plastic mask was nauseating.

My asthmatic children would always cry and fight when we placed the plastic masks over their faces. The medicine delivered by the mask was supposed to make them feel better, but the noise, the strange smell of the mask, and their lack of understanding made them afraid of the procedure. Having a stranger hold them down and put something over their face was terrifying. Since my asthma symptoms are often accompanied by a sensation of claustrophobia, I can identify with their terror.

I have decided to take the anti-fungal medicine again. Doctor I1 had advised me to stop taking it the night I was admitted to emergency, but now that my symptoms are receding, I'm anxious to resume my treatment. Doctor ID1, in Memphis, had indicated that I should take the medication for a year. I break all the rules and swallow the pill without telling the nurse.

I'm regretting my hasty decision. My limbs are slowly losing function. The nausea is coming in waves. Is it the anti-fungal medication that is slowly poisoning me?

The nurse has given me an anti-nausea pill. Through my drugged state, half sleep and half consciousness, I'm aware of the crushing sensation in my chest. Cold and numbness pervade my agitated body. I toss and turn, shifting positions again and again, my mind in a state of total confusion. I need to tell Mom, but Mom's not here. Where am I? I'm in a hospital. I should call the nurse. I can't; my arms are too heavy to reach the bell. It's such an effort to breathe. Something is poisoning me, but I'm just too tired to deal with it.

**December 7**

No more anti-nausea medicine for me. Feeling drugged during an episode is worse than facing it with my mind intact. I can wait for my waves of sickness to pass. I have managed this far. No more anti-fungal medicine either. I'll wait until I have instructions to continue since last night proved these medications create more problems than they solve.

Grace and I are discussing Doctor I1's suggestion that all my symptoms could be caused by Crohn's disease. Since I had learned to live with the constant stomach aches, I hadn't emphasized this condition to the doctors. My test in Memphis had revealed nothing, so there had been no reason for Doctor G1 to conduct further research. Does Crohn's disease produce such a wide range of symptoms?

Apparently the results from my spinal tap and bone marrow tests in Memphis showed white blood cells in the spinal fluid and elevated white cells in the bone marrow. Doctor N2 wants to conduct another spinal tap. Why had I not been given this information by Doctor N1?

Now that I'm feeling slightly better, I'm anxious to leave the hospital. My room affords little privacy, particularly now that a new roommate has joined us. Her huge family fills the room during visiting hours and their chatting and laughing definitely cuts into my afternoon nap time. However, the worst part of the scenario plays between one and four in the morning. During her sleep, this woman continually coughs and expectorates phlegm, which is accompanied by much passing of wind at a less than delicate volume. Unfortunately for me, I'm not deaf or semiconscious like my other roommates.

Doctor N2 chats with me as he sets up the tray for the lumbar puncture, his conversation conveying a genuine concern for my plight. Although he understands the financial burden of my escalating hospital bills, he thinks I should remain in the hospital until the doctors find a solution to my problem. His words run through my mind as I cling to the bed rail, gritting my teeth against the force of the needle.

## December 8

The pattern continues, but I feel well enough to leave the hospital and continue my investigation at home. Apparently my sputum test has indicated fungus. Doctor I1 is making arrangements for me to see an infectious disease specialist at another hospital in the city, one who has studied his specialty in Texas. I'm elated as I know he'll be very well acquainted with my problem.

## December 10

There is only one bedroom, so I've encamped in the living room of the apartment, with the ocean and mountains just outside my window and my few belongings scattered around the TV and sofa. Unfortunately, the view is wasted on me, as I spend my waking hours thinking of ways to improve my health.

Nothing has changed, better when I first wake up, sickest during the late evening and early morning. Mom still has to assist me to the bathroom and shower. My ten day holiday has been spent in a cramped hospital ward. The return portion of my ticket reads December 10th, but Memphis will have to wait some time to celebrate my return.

Mom still insists that food and the timing of my episodes are related.

"Heather, we have to develop a strategy to beat this problem. If we were trying to find a solution to a business problem, we would find every piece of available information to help us solve it. How can this be any different? Search back in your mind. When did you start having problems?"

"I started to have asthma attacks and fatigue shortly after I moved to San Antonio. Remember I was ill last year on my birthday with that flu. I couldn't seem to get better for a long time and dragged myself to work for months."

"Did you eat differently in San Antonio than you did in New Orleans?"

"Yes, I started to eat a lot of beef and corn tortillas." I had changed my eating habits when I moved to San Antonio. Maybe avoiding beef will help.

**December 15**

The rain pummels against the window of the car. Pedestrians scuttle home, their umbrellas like shields against the forces of nature. As I lie in the back of the car, gathering strength for the appointment, chills rack my body.

# The Toxic Labyrinth

It's apparent that I can't make it up several floors to the doctor's office, even with Mom's supportive arm. A wheelchair presents the only alternative. I sit, clutching the arms of the chair, my head drooping on my lap.

I lean my head against the wall of the waiting room, listening to Mom make arrangements with the receptionist. The fluorescent lights illuminate the white walls. Medical offices are always so harsh, never soothing. Flu-like symptoms wash over me. I close my eyes searching for a few minutes of relief.

Mom hands the doctor my file. Is all that paper about me? I used to be one outdated sheet in some doctor's file. I welcome the rest on the examining table while he reads the contents. What's he asking me? Everything is so foggy. My body shivers from the pervasive cold that never seems to leave. Mom covers me with her coat to keep me warm.

According to Doctor ID2, I don't have fungus. I'm too ill to ask any questions, but I understand the important part. No more medication. What a relief! Doctor ID1 in Memphis had warned me that the medication would have to be delivered directly into my heart by IV, if the oral dosage didn't work. Maybe all my symptoms are related to my Crohn's after all.

Back home, Mom and I discuss my previous bout with Crohn's seven years ago. Some of the symptoms I experienced then were similar, but not nearly as severe. At that time, I spent five days on clear fluids and improved enough to return to work after a few weeks.

We decide to try a liquid diet for a few days. Because my condition escalates five to six hours after I have eaten, this strategy should give us some information. It will be our plan of action, until my January appointment with my former gastroenterologist, Doctor G2.

**December 16**

An improvement in my health! I've slept through the night. The diet of apple juice, water, chicken soup, and gelatin may be working.

It's evening and I can get to the bathroom unaided. I pray we've found the answer.

**December 17**

More progress. For the first time since I arrived home, I can navigate the stairs. It's time to venture outdoors for a few hours. Mom is having lunch with a former student from her days as junior high school teacher and I'm going to join them. At the restaurant, the three of us laugh and reminisce. Even though I can't partake of the food, I can enjoy visiting in a normal setting.

**December 18**

Mom and I take a short, slow walk within the confines of the neighborhood to buy me my own crystal for Christmas. Because she is terribly afraid of flying, Mom needs her good luck crystal before leaving on her trip to Los Angeles. Besides, she thinks it's time I had one of my own.

Not only have I walked the whole distance to the shop, I've scaled the flight of stairs to the second floor. The room contains a wealth of crystal designs, from intricate sculptures to tiny pendants. We choose a clear octagon on a silver ring as my good health charm. To complete the ritual, we walk to the sea which washes against the rocks just behind Mom's apartment. She takes my crystal, dips it into the water, and hangs it around my neck, willing its strength to bring me good health. I take Mom's crystal, place it around her neck, and give her a hug. It's good to be home.

# The Toxic Labyrinth

## December 19

Was it just four days ago that I was in the wheelchair? I walk up the long hill, the fresh scent of the ocean adding to my well being. My Crohn's has settled down. The nausea has disappeared. Tomorrow I'll add solid food to my menu.

Mom insists on decorating the apartment for Don and me before she leaves on her Christmas holiday, and has persuaded me to come shopping for a tree. We walk around the lot, discussing the attributes of those trees in our price range. A small pine, just the right size for the apartment leans against a wall of larger trees. We purchase our symbol of the season, stuff it in the trunk of the car, and head for home.

The tree is obviously meant for me. Beside the sofa, it stands slightly crooked in the stand, bringing its own special warmth to my small corner of the world.

## December 20

The solid food is healing my body. For the first time since September, my left arm is starting to feel normal. The pain and numbness are fading.

Only three more sleeps before Don arrives for our first Christmas together. Unfortunately, some of the Christmas presents I bought are gathering dust in my Memphis apartment.

## December 21

Mom and Doug have left for their Christmas holiday, so Dad has agreed to stay with me until Don arrives.

Shopping for a new dress, my Christmas present from Dad, is a revelation. I try on numerous outfits, but nothing fits. The weight I've gained over the past year taunts me from the mirror of every dressing room. Attempting to shoehorn my current form into a size ten is an exercise in futility. Is there no piece of clothing that doesn't emphasize my figure in the wrong places?

I'm miserable, hungry, and grumpy. Will Don notice my weight gain? Once more I look in the mirror, expecting to be disappointed. The wonders that a basic black dress can perform. A slim, elegant woman is reflected in the glass. Let the Yuletide season begin!

## December 23

Don grabs me in a big bear hug. We laugh and chat during the drive from the airport. The old sociable me is back. Now that I have the answer, Christmas will be fun.

## December 25

The ceremonial mask stares at me from the box. A brass figure of a woman, carrying a child at her hip, stands on the table. Christmas presents from Nigeria. The present from Jean nestles in layers of tissue paper. Elegantly covered with cream lace and pink roses, the jewelry box is perfect for the dresser of my Victorian dream house.

Most of the treasures I have accumulated during my travels line the walls and shelves of Mom's apartment, waiting for me to find a permanent home. My Christmas presents will join the ranks of this expanding craft collection.

Don and I talk about our future plans and my return to Memphis. Once the Christmas season is over, I should be able to resume my life there again.

After a few phone calls to Mom in Los Angeles, I am ready to serve my first Christmas dinner to Don and Dad. Just a little turkey and potato for me. Don is home. I'm cured. It doesn't matter that I can't eat my usual portion of food.

# The Toxic Labyrinth

## December 26

The last few days have been wonderful. Without the constant symptoms, I have been able to enjoy the Christmas season.

Chinatown in Vancouver is a wonderful experience of sights and smells: sidewalk stalls overflowing with exotic vegetables, spicy aromas wafting from the numerous restaurants, shops filled with strange herbs, roots, and plants.

This is Don's first visit to Vancouver and his tour won't be complete without sampling Chinese dining at its finest. I join in with a small plate of dim sum. Just a taste, as spicy food is not recommended for people with Crohn's.

## December 27

The rain has ceased for a few days, bringing clear blue skies and freshly washed air. My slight headache—a symptom that I'll ignore—is not going to impede Don's continuing tour of Vancouver sights. We have a great day filled with laughter. Seeing a city with someone you love brings a fresh perspective to well-known landmarks. It's wonderful to be in love. Fresh pasta and clams for supper. Why not? This very bland food should be no problem.

## December 28

My face feels strange and my head aches. No matter, I don't have the time to waste on these minor symptoms.

Don and I really missed eating seafood when we lived in the US heartland. Tonight we plan a lobster dinner with Dad, our west coast treat. As we read the cooking instructions, assemble the tools, and set the table, the anticipated feast of lobster and pasta fuels our hunger.

After dinner my symptoms return with such a vengeance that the discomfort in my hips is restricting movement. The cause has to be the lobster, but this doesn't make sense because the meal was so bland. Don rubs my back to soothe the pain until I manage to fall asleep.

**December 29**

Returning to the limited diet of clear fluids will help rest my bowel and give me relief from the constant symptoms. I have obtained a prescription for the medicine I had taken when I was first diagnosed with Crohn's. Should I take it? Seven years ago the doctor told me the medication was optional, and because it had not relieved my stomach aches, I stopped taking it after a few weeks. Maybe my condition is more advanced this time, and it'll work.

Even the small amount of water that I drink is uncomfortable to swallow. Don lies on the bed with me. I'm not feeling well enough to move around, so we play board games and talk.

Tonight I've made a special effort to attend a play, in honor of Mom's return from Los Angeles. During the performance, my concentration is interrupted constantly by agitation and chest pains. The white gas, part of the dry ice stage effects, wafts through the audience. The crushing sensation in my chest makes me want to scream out.

**December 30**

Thirst invades my body, but drinking water is a problem when I can't swallow. The pressure in my chest is intense. The dulling cold is back, accompanied by the flu-like feeling and numbness in my left arm.

Don has discovered the medical library on Internet. If I can't go to the library to do research, Mom's computer will allow me to search for answers at home. We roam the health data base, looking for articles on Crohn's. Bland food appears to be the correct choice for my condition, although shellfish are rated high on the list of foods to be avoided. That explains why my symptoms are back. Lobster and clams must be eliminated from my diet. We're on the right track.

**December 31**

I have never missed a New Year's Eve celebration since I was old enough to walk. Don has purchased tickets for a dinner and dance, ensuring that this year will be no exception.

My condition is not improving as the day progresses. Don suggests that we stay home, but I'm not going to miss the evening's festivities. So what, if I can't eat or drink, I just have to get there. Attributing my weakness to my much reduced diet, I lie on the couch, gathering energy until it's time to dress.

As I walk up the stairs to the nightclub, I look down at my feet. Are they attached to my legs? Strangely, I can't feel my shoes.

Apple juice is not on the bar menu, leaving water as my only drink option. Don doesn't want to eat in front of me. I assure him there's no point in wasting his food ticket. Although I appear to converse with friends, my thoughts are scattered and my brain tries to field the disjointed phrases of conversation. It's only 10:30. How much longer can I keep this up? For the first time in my life, a band is playing, and I don't have the energy or will to dance. I attract Don's attention and signal my intention to leave.

At home, the warmth of the sofa comforts me. My symptoms are abating. I'm just tired. That explains my problems.

# CHAPTER 5

## BLIND ALLEYS

Each path is a blind alley leading me deeper into the maze.

# The Toxic Labyrinth

## 1994

### January 1

The ball drops in Times Square. The year is behind me and not a minute too soon. I've never greeted the New Year watching TV. My reputation as the party queen is being seriously challenged. But I think we're on the right track. Shouldn't be long before I'm celebrating a new beginning of my own.

Mom and Doug are having their usual New Year's Day gathering. The highlight of the evening takes place when the guests read their predictions from the past year and make new ones for the coming year.

How I love to be social, to explore the world around me through another person's thoughts. Rob, a former junior high school teacher, and I exchange news and reminisce about school pranks. In the background, I hear Don entertaining those around him with tales of Nigeria.

The predictions will be made without me. The party is over for me much too soon. I have remained on clear fluids for the day, and my weakened body can't last until the guests depart. Don and I discretely leave the party for the quiet of the bedroom.

Whenever he has the opportunity, Don sits at Mom's computer retrieving medical articles. He enjoys this focus, a project that gives him a purpose and something to fill the long hours when I'm confined indoors. To take my mind off the sounds of the party filtering into the bedroom, Don brings out a folder of articles on Crohn's disease and suggests we read them together. Understanding the effects of this disease will help him solve this problem that confronts us. It's comforting to know that he's here for me and interested in finding the answers. How can I not love him?

What a finish to New Year's Day, a bed covered with medical articles on bowel disorders.

**January 2**

I've tried so hard to cope, but I can barely swallow. So far, I've managed only a small glass of water during the day. My body will fail, if I can't eat. Maybe a vitamin pill will give me temporary nutrition until my body permits me to eat.

A major mistake, the vitamin pill has made me extremely ill; it has brought back all my symptoms with a vengeance: nausea, joint pains, inability to swallow, and a crushing sensation in my chest that leaves me gasping for breath. The retching has forced me into a decision to go to the emergency room. I'm too sick to wait the two days until my appointment with Doctor G2. Because I'm still on my American health care plan until February, I worry about the cost of another emergency room visit and possible hospitalization. Don dismisses my worries by saying my health is more important than the cost. Doug prepares the car, Mom dresses me, and Don carries me, because I'm too weak to walk; a family outing to the emergency room.

This is the fourth institution—counting emergency room visits—in the growing list of hospitals I've known and loved. Doctor G2 works here, giving me no choice, but to start the process all over again.

Everything is happening in slow motion. Can my legs, these two columns of jelly, hold me long enough for the nurse to take a standing blood pressure?

"She's dehydrated." The nurse's words penetrate my haze. What does she want? I'm too sick to care. Don is beside me and can handle things.

New hospital, same old routine of vital signs, blood samples, and IV. These activities swirl around me, drawing me deeper into the role of patient, while my days as a caregiver become distant memories. The IV nurse places the tourniquet around my arm and slaps my hand to locate a vein. What's happening? I can't feel my hands. My hands have been numb before, never lifeless. This sensation progresses to my elbows, and soon my feet experience the same loss of feeling.

"Don, I can't feel my hands! I can't move them."

"Relax," the IV nurse replies calmly. "You're just nervous about the IV."

"I'm used to getting an IV. I've had lots of experience lately."

My body is sending a clear signal that something is wrong. The IV nurse poises the catheter and stabs the vein in my hand. The blood is supposed to flow into the IV catheter immediately, but the vein is in complete spasm. Panicked, Don calls out to a nurse passing by my cubicle. The blood finally flows from the IV catheter, and I watch the solution infuse, as rapidly as possible, into my vein. The other nurse, alerted by Don's outburst, has returned with medication and instructs me to take it.

"What are you giving me?" I ask.

"A relaxant."

"I'm not anxious. I've no sensation in my hands." Obediently, I put the medicine under my tongue and stifle any more remarks.

Don is holding my hand. I can't sense his grip or squeeze his hand. Each minute that passes marks my inability to feel my hands and legs, as well as the continuing loss of control over my body. The worry on Don's face reveals his concern. He knows my condition is not caused by stress and anxiety.

The IV fluid infuses into my vein, replacing the numbing cold with a soothing warmth. Even though I'm still weak and my hands haven't regained complete function, I can squeeze Don's hand, a definite turn for the better in my world of so few victories. He gives me a hug. "Your hands were ice cold when you were complaining about the lack of sensation. After you said the feeling was returning, I could feel your hands become warm in mine."

God, please don't take Don away from me. I need him beside me, if I'm going to fight this demon. I'm so afraid of what is to come.

**January 3**

It's after midnight. A bag of IV fluid, a room on the ward, and a tranquil body give me hope for tomorrow. The bedside curtain protects us from prying eyes, as Don whispers assuring words quietly in the dark and gives me many kisses good-bye. When he leaves I cry silently. It's distressing to miss even one of our few nights together.

A nurse gathering the usual admission information has replaced Don at my bedside. A loud complaint issues from the other side of the bed curtain. Words of welcome from my new roommate? The nurse looks at me and announces loudly that she is almost finished.

The loud snoring emanating from the next bed convinces me that the conversation hadn't disturbed my roommate's sleep. The IV is comforting, no worries about what to drink or eat. Lying awake and listening to the routine hospital sounds, I think about the reversal of my role and wonder whether I will ever be the nurse on the night shift again.

The thin rays of morning struggle to light my corner of the ward, as Doctor G2 pushes back the curtain on his rounds. It's apparent that he's not happy to see me. "Why are you in the hospital?"

"I'm having trouble swallowing," I explain.

Doctor G2 is unimpressed. After remarking that I have to eat, he leaves the room without taking a history. Why am I on trial? I remember this doctor to be a personable man. What has changed? My stubborn nature reasserts itself while I think about his last comment. First, I'll use the IV to help my body settle down and then I'll eat when I'm good and ready.

From behind the protection of the bed curtain, my unsociable roommate loudly announces to her doctor that she hasn't slept because of the noise in the middle of the night. I want to point out it was probably the roar of her snoring that kept her awake. What a production over five minutes of lost sleep. I won't be drawing back the privacy curtain to make her acquaintance.

Ensconced in my cubical, curtain drawn, headphones plugged in, I quietly watch the nine o'clock TV show. The call bell from the next bed has summoned the nurse. My roommate insists she can't sleep with the roar of the TV in her ears. The nurse steps to my side of the curtain and asks if I've heard the complaint.

"Yes, I'll turn off the TV," I reply.

I grab my IV pole and stride to the other side of the curtain. "Why didn't you ask me to turn off the TV instead of ringing the nurse?" I inquire.

"I'm so sick."

"This is a hospital. You're not the only one. We're all sick."

## January 4

The annoying voice rises from the other bed. My roommate is complaining again to her doctor about her sleepless night. What a crock this is. Her snoring entertained me for hours after I shut off the TV. The doctor commiserates and promises to arrange for a private room to reduce her stress. It's important for her to concentrate on getting well. He'll also fill out a request form, stating a private room is required for medical reasons, so she won't have to pay extra for the privilege. What nonsense! Don and I were told no private rooms were available. We obviously didn't understand the way the system works.

The resident, studying to be a gastroenterologist, is friendly and wants to take a lengthy history, so I dredge up all the facts. I mention that food is definitely a factor in my illness. The flu-like feeling, pain, and numbness have receded on the fluid diet. He asks whether eating green vegetables increases my asthma, and I tell him I haven't noticed any relation. Next, his questioning turns to what he considers the area of greatest concern, the numbness and tingling. He will arrange for a neurologist to see me. I protest that nothing will show up on the tests. Since I've already been prodded and poked by two neurologists, I'm not interested in seeing another one, but he insists and I lose.

**January 5**

Even though Doctor N3, the neurologist, appears caring and considerate, I'm disinterested in this meeting. What will he find that's different? The numbness and the occasional loss of my grasp concern him, so he tests my strength. Again my left side is much weaker. He dismisses this by noting I'm right handed. As I explain that my left side isn't always this weak, he shakes his head, suggesting that he doesn't agree with me, and mentions the possibility of multiple sclerosis. I repeat that all my numbness disappears when I stop eating and that my condition is related to food, not MS.

My new roommates are young, but their conditions give me no confidence in my own future. Both are battling chronic diseases which are eating away energy and body substance, a little bit at a time. June, who has Crohn's, has been sentenced to a life revolving around hospital care; Bev is yellow and cries in pain from the ravages of liver disease.

**January 6**

I'm making progress, as each day brings my body much closer to normal. However, another TB test looms before me. Even though I was checked in Memphis, there's a chance I could have TB in my intestine.

While preparing to inject me, the nurse announces that she really doesn't remember how to administer a TB test. As she starts toward me with the bevel of the needle pointed downward, I remind her that it has to point upward in order to make the small bubble under my skin. Nervously, she laughs at her mistake and stabs the skin, driving the needle too deep. What can I do? I just pray the procedure will be over quickly.

Soon the left side of my throat is closing and the nausea, a crushing sensation in my chest, and violent shaking add to my distress. This reaction, identical to the one I had experienced after the TB test in Memphis, wracks my body. I ring the nurse and request medication for the nausea. The left side of my throat continues to swell, and I throw up into the basin by my bed, trying to gag quietly so I don't disturb my roommates. Interesting that the reaction has affected only the left side of my throat, even though my right arm was injected.

**January 7**

Sick for most of the night, I am angry because the test has made me ill, just when I was beginning to feel normal. The flu-like feeling has returned, so I'm awake and retching when the doctors come by on rounds. Even though I explain the events of yesterday evening, they dismiss my remark, saying that no one reacts to the TB test in that manner.

"But I've had the test many times before with no reaction. For some reason, something has changed." Ignoring my comments, they decide to order a pregnancy test. Are they joking?

"I'm not pregnant." My protests are ignored.

When the dietitian visited me to discuss increasing my nutritional intake, she suggested protein gelatin and a liquid food. Because it makes me gag, I refused the liquid food. The smell of it reminds me of administering this supplement through a feeding tube to patients too debilitated to care for themselves. The protein gelatin is not much more appealing, but I'm confident I can tolerate it better.

No reactions from the tests for candida and mumps. Despite what the doctors thought, I *had* reacted to the TB test.

Doctor G2 has ordered an upper GI test for Monday. I protested that I wasn't ready, but I have no bargaining power. How will I swallow the barium mixture, a task that is difficult enough when I feel healthy? At least I have two days to prepare.

**January 9**

Don visits faithfully every day. We lie on the bed, sharing the earphones, one ear piece each, and watch TV. We read my book on bowel disorders and design special diets for my condition. (My hospital trays are not prepared for someone with Crohn's disease.) Instead of a hospital gown, I wear the T-shirt and ball cap Don has bought me, and this restores some semblance of normality to my life. He takes me for short walks outside, down the hall, to the cafeteria, any diversion from the confinement of this room.

I vent my frustrations to him. "No one is listening to me. When will I be myself again?" I break down and cry, because I can't bear to be sick any longer. Listening patiently, Don tells me he loves me and dries my tears.

I want to go home. We're spending most of his leave in the hospital, our freedom restricted by this monster that holds me captive. The time for his departure is drawing closer, but I don't even want to think about that.

**January 10**

How will I swallow the little gas pills and chalky barium? I take the large cup in my hands and peer at the seemingly bottomless contents. Although my stomach has ingested only clear fluids for the past week, I'll do my best to drink this elixir from hell, a mixture thick and unpleasant. I drink, I retch, but I'm determined to succeed. I'm not going through these preliminaries again. I swallow faster.

# The Toxic Labyrinth

Whatever starts to come back up my throat, I swallow again while my mind focuses on returning home and spending time with Don.

It is now five hours since the test. All my symptoms have returned, and I wait for the shaking to subside. My problem must be connected to what goes into my digestive system. The results of my upper GI series have to show something.

## January 11

Nothing! The test has revealed nothing! There is a limited section of my small intestine that shows a slight patchwork appearance, a finding that doesn't require medication or account for my symptoms.

I've started to eat small amounts of solid food. The 'BRAT' diet, one that is used by Crohn's patients to settle the bowel, will be my fare for the next while. Mom brings the menu of banana, rice, applesauce, and toast to the hospital every day. I eat only the food she prepares. That way we know for certain what I'm eating. So far, I seem to be tolerating the regimen. Maybe my body will settle down on its own, and I can leave the hospital before I have to endure more useless tests.

The nurse announces I'm scheduled for release after an eye test for MS and a spinal tap. Spinal tap!! No way, no more of those. I'm going to refuse. The two I've had are enough to last a life time. Once the eye test is completed, I intend to disappear before Doctor N3 can find me to do the spinal tap.

Sitting for two hours in this chair with flu-like symptoms assaulting me makes concentration on the black and white dots almost impossible. This test is giving me a headache. Now they tell me I've been concentrating on the wrong dot. The screen is covered with dots. How am I supposed to know which dot is the important one? My mind doesn't want to center on dots any more. I want to lie down, not repeat part of this test. The next wave of nausea emphasizes my thoughts.

The tray for the dreaded spinal tap mocks me from the bedside table. Don confirms my suspicions that Doctor N3 has been to my room while I was out having the eye test. We have to escape.

As a parting gift, the nurse has given me an injection in my left leg. The abnormally long clotting times in my blood work may indicate a lack of vitamin K. Barely able to put pressure on my leg, I lean on Don as we walk down the corridor.

Home to Mom's, a place with food and no injections. I smile with satisfaction as I climb into the car, knowing I've escaped the spinal tap. My symptoms return as the car moves toward home. When I start to cry, Don asks if he should take me back to the hospital.

"I'm not going back. What's the sense in returning to the hospital? The doctors don't listen to me." I have to pull myself together, to put on a brave face for Don.

I climb into bed. The vitamin shot has made my leg burn and my hips ache. Since we have no hot water bottle, Don heats water in a glass jar and massages my leg with the warmth until I fall asleep.

**January 12**

My leg has improved. I've graduated to more solid food: tofu, bananas, pasta, bread, and eggs. I'm trying to eat as much protein as I can while still maintaining my bland diet.

We have to accomplish as much as we can while I'm feeling well. Don will be returning to Africa in five days. As we stroll down the street toward the theater, the promise of an exciting evening pushes everything else from my mind. The lounge resonates with the sound of casual conversation. Waiting in line for the theater doors to open, patrons discuss the merits of the play. I sit, drinking in the atmosphere, reveling in my night on the town like a child on Christmas morning. We seat ourselves at the back of the theater since I breathe more easily where the crowd is sparse.

# The Toxic Labyrinth

A stroll up Robson Street after the play. The smell of espresso makes me crave its taste. Watching the diners laugh and enjoy after theater drinks and dinner, I wonder when I'll be a part of this scene again.

We retrace our steps to the car. Suddenly, my hands won't close, I'm dizzy, and my surroundings appear hazy. I clutch at Don's arm for support knowing that the parking lot is two blocks away. Can I make it? With each step my ice cold feet drag along the sidewalk, even though I command them to walk. I look at my watch, 10:45 p.m., exactly six hours since I ate my dinner of salad and pasta.

When we arrive home, Don carries me to the shower and turns on the hot water to soothe my pains. The aching in my hip joints makes standing difficult, and he supports me while the hot water caresses the unbearable aches. After helping me out of the shower, Don hugs me and tucks me into bed. I start to cry. Nothing I try is working. Why can't my body let me enjoy the few short days we have together before he leaves?

**January 14**

Mom's apartment does not afford much privacy. I've convinced Don that a short weekend trip is the treat we owe ourselves for these last few days together. Don insists on staying close to the city, and we have compromised. Our destination is a bed and breakfast on Bowen Island, a twenty-minute ferry ride away.

Before we leave, I take some of the medicine I purchased earlier for my Crohn's to reduce any inflammation and ensure that I have a symptom-free two days on the island. On our way out of the apartment I glance at my reflection in the mirror, at the very pale and much thinner me. Must be the ten pounds I lost while I was in the hospital. I'm down to one hundred and fifty pounds.

The weather is beautiful, but cool. The ferry skims across the open water. Mountains to the north invite skiers to enjoy their snow capped peaks. Sea birds dart between the ferry and land, leading us toward our destination. I huddle in the warmth of Don's arms, our bodies braced against the brisk breeze. We laugh. A special time. We're going to have fun, just the two of us. Bowen Island comes into view, a small piece of land squatting on the water, its rocky terrain blanketed with conifers.

For us the bed and breakfast lacks character. We're used to old southern mansions, furnished with antiques and civil war memorabilia. Despite this, the house is a monumental improvement over my hospital accommodations. The hostess appears disinterested in answering our questions about the area, and so we must discover any points of interest on our own. Off we go to find the craft stores.

I love shopping for crafts, my favorite pastime when I travel. After looking around the store, I have to sit down for a break. The flu-like symptoms still plague me and have quickly sapped my energy.

The restaurant overlooks the picturesque bay. Sailboats moored in the marina are silhouetted against the darkening sky. Although the menu lists a variety of tempting dishes, I resist and order plain, boiled noodles. I try to enjoy the meal, but the intermittent periods of sickness are defeating me. Don mustn't know. He's having such a good time.

My sluggish legs want only to rest. If I concentrate, I should make it back to our lodgings without alarming Don, especially since he didn't want to travel this far from the city and instant medical assistance.

The hot tub relaxes and limbers up my joints. I have taken more medicine, so that is probably helping as well. My relaxed state activates the hunger button, and I eat the remains of the pasta from my doggie bag. Immersed in the hot water, Don and I plan. Now that I'm out of the hospital, where do we go from here? Do I return to Memphis and if so, when? With Don flying to Africa on Monday, there is a great deal to discuss. I hug him and whisper that I'll miss him. His leaving is even more difficult to bear when my life is so uncertain.

**January 15**

My eyes fly open. I can't breathe, and the crushing chest pains leave me gasping for air. Clutching the sides of the toilet bowl, I retch and retch. I'm cold and every joint aches, yet my nerves are burning. Don holds my hair away from my face and rubs my back. With each wave of nausea, I pray for the sickness to cease. I had wanted so much for our last few days together to be special.

My body is shaking, washing away the sickness with each tremor. For two hours I've been crouched over the toilet, and finally I can lean back to rest against Don. We sit together on the cold bathroom tile, my sickness abated for the moment.

Sore and aching, I drag my body into bed. Did the pasta make me sick? It's exactly six hours since I ate the first helping at the restaurant. If pasta is the culprit, I'll know in another hour. I polished off the second helping in the hot tub. Exhausted, I slumber for just forty-five minutes before the second helping of pasta adds to my misery. To make matters worse, this time my lower end decides to get into the act, and I retch into a bucket while sitting on the toilet. A new development surfaces, blood passes from my bowel. The large clots, bright red pools floating among the effluent, add their own emphasis to my plight.

I climb back into bed with the four hours of continuous retching behind me. My side hurts and my teeth chatter as I shake with the cold. Under the skin, my nerves burn like hot brands. Don lies beside me, holding my depleted body, his body language conveying his worry. We decide to catch the first ferry in the morning.

Why will no one listen when I relate my symptoms to food? I can set my watch by these reactions. The night of the play I experienced numb hands and feet, a flu-like feeling during my walk to the car. I'd eaten pasta that night, too. I doze intermittently, waking frequently to look at my watch. I don't want to miss the first ferry.

Don helps me pack and dress for the trip home, relieved that he didn't give in to my wishes of a more distant location for our trip.

Back in our living room abode, I dive under the inviting warmth of the covers, comforted by the security and familiarity of this room. But I have to eat something. Maybe a boiled egg will be safe. A bad decision. The egg is causing me to retch and throw up so violently my stomach feels like it's coming through my face. My body is telling me I have no choice, but to return to the hospital. We reactivate the family emergency room response. Don carries me in his arms, because I'm too weak to walk. I've lost my strength.

Doctor ER2—the list of people connected to my care is growing—listens to my well rehearsed history. I add that every time I eat pasta, I become very ill. He shrugs his shoulders in response. After I emphasize that clots of blood are issuing from my bowel, he does order an x-ray of my abdomen to check for a blockage.

The expected scenario is unfolding; two large bags of IV fluid and I'm starting to recover. Why does my blood work indicate dehydration? I have been drinking juice and water constantly to alleviate my persistent thirst.

Don holds my hand and makes jokes. He strokes my hair, each stroke expressing how much he loves and needs me. There's no doubt in his mind we'll find the solution, the cure. The doctors will listen, now that we have proof of my problem with food. Surely they have tests to check out this theory.

We have requested a private room, but only a semi-private is available. It's Saturday evening and Don leaves Monday afternoon. The understanding nurse grants our wish to be together and allows Don to sit in my room for the night. He sits in a chair by the bed, holding my hand while I sleep.

# The Toxic Labyrinth

Sleep is fitful. I wake up to ensure that my IV is dripping. Each time the nurse hangs a new bag of IV fluid, I wait until she leaves, then standing on my bed, I read the label to make sure I'm receiving the correct solution. I'm losing confidence in my hospital treatment. How do I maintain control? Am I a difficult patient? No, I'm just being cautious.

## January 16

Our last day together. I always seem to land in the hospital about the time Don leaves: October, December, and now January. How I want him to stay. I know I'm luckier than most women. When he is home from Nigeria, we can spend so much time together.

I'm not ready to walk any distance yet. Don pushes me in the wheelchair to the hospital cafeteria for our last evening together. Fifteen minutes is all I last before I have to return to the room. The retching begins as I'm crawling into bed. To supplement what little nutrition I'm receiving these days, I swallowed a vitamin pill on the way to the cafeteria. Is the retching and nausea the result of this?

"Do you want something to settle your stomach," the nurse asks.

"Yes, I want a pill."

She looks perplexed. "Putting the medication in your IV is simpler. Especially when you're nauseated and retching."

A logical solution, but I refuse. I want to see the medicine before I take it. Maintaining control is important.

Visiting hours are over, but Don disregards the announcement and pulls a small, gaily wrapped package from his pocket.

"Happy Birthday."

Soon it will be my thirty-first birthday. Will I be celebrating in this cubicle hooked to an IV? The gold humming bird, symbolic for its healing powers, shines in its cotton bed. Taking the necklace from the box, Don hangs it around my neck.

"For luck," he whispers.

Don gives me many hugs good-bye. Each time he leaves, I fear that I'll never see him again. I pray nothing happens to him in Nigeria as it is a dangerous country. He kisses me for the last time and is gone.

**January 17**

The gastroenterology team stands at the foot of my bed and announces that more aggressive testing is in order. They'll actually look inside my bowel this time. Will this test prove that my condition is caused by food? My recovery on IV fluids is speedier than during my previous January hospital visit. Already I've started drinking clear fluids.

Rich, entertaining as ever, sits on the edge of my bed and spins stories that briefly divert my attention to the world outside this institution. A close friend since he was my zoology lab instructor at university, he always delights in pointing out that I attended his Friday lab at my convenience, when Wednesday beer night took priority over his early Thursday morning lab.

**January 18**

The sigmoidoscopy, a test that uses a special scope to look at the last segment of the large bowel, can detect if there are any areas of bleeding or disease. It's much more exact than an x-ray.

A few months after I was diagnosed with Crohn's disease, I made arrangements to travel to the Virgin Islands. Wanting reassurance that my condition would not create a problem during my travels, I had Doctor G2 perform this test prior to my departure. The test had revealed nothing of concern.

My memories of the first sigmoidoscopy are still vivid. The instructional pamphlet did not fully prepare me for circumstances

# The Toxic Labyrinth

where I had to bare my bottom to a male nurse. It was embarrassing enough to reveal my derriere to a male doctor, but the male nurse was more than I had bargained for.

That test involved a very small scope. This time I'm in for a large surprise, no pun intended. The scope looks awfully long and thick. No message of comfort here. I close my eyes and clench my teeth, visions of that first test all too clear in my mind. As I thought, the procedure has not improved over the past five years. Unfortunately, the only scenery in my bowel is provided by chunks of old barium from the test the week before. We're no further ahead.

Because my pains are much higher up in the region of the small bowel, I really want the doctors to look at my small bowel with a scope, but instead I'm scheduled for a barium enema. I'm not delighted at the prospect of more barium in my body, and the location of delivery isn't my first choice either.

The nurse hands me the two page instruction sheet, a two day preparation of clear fluids and laxatives preceding the test. The laxatives come in a variety of forms, the repulsive drinks and the more subtle pill. Why two days, if I'm consuming mainly clear fluids? Apparently, all patients prepare for two days, regardless of diet. Clear fluids for all meals and laxatives for dessert.

## January 19

The student tech is preparing for me. Does someone contrive to have male assistants for me when I'm having embarrassing and invasive tests? The large bag of barium confirms that it won't be an easy day. I lie on the table, behind exposed with a tube dangling out the end. What are they announcing? The radiologist is being paged repeatedly over the loud speaker. Cinderella's ready for the ball and they're paging the Prince.

Twenty-five minutes later he finally arrives. Was he in hiding? Had he discovered that his first morning case was a barium enema? Except for the fact that I have this piece of tubing the size of a garden hose extending out my back end, I wouldn't have cared about his late appearance. However, the keen tech had me strapped up and ready to go the minute I rolled into the testing room.

The more barium that pours in, the more my discomfort level rises. I'm instructed to rotate on the table while they observe the bowel from different angles on the x-ray images. I have to perform this feat attached to an IV pole with a hose protruding from my behind. These pleasures are enhanced each time I bang the IV tube against the table and move the catheter in my hand.

Step right up folks! See Heather, the star of our show, perform her balancing act. She's clamped to the testing table, an IV in one hand, a tube jutting out of her curvaceous bottom, and two bags of barium up her gut.

When the radiologist pumps air through the tube into my bowel, the pain is excruciating. Two hours of this torture to endure, before I can return to my room. The procedure hurts so much, I bang the pillow with my fist. Do I care who sees me cry at this point? I have been looking at the last four months through a veil of tears. Something involving this much pain has to lead to an answer.

**January 20**

I have begun to eat again, half an egg, a gourmet treat to one who is starved for the taste of anything that is not liquid. If I start out slowly, maybe my body will accept the small, bland meals without making me ill. Convinced there's a problem with my bowel, even though no one believes me, I've decided to keep a diary to show the doctor the relationship between the food I'm eating and any subsequent symptoms.

Doctor N3 has discovered I'm back in residence. Referring to my avoidance of the spinal tap during my last hospitalization, he makes it clear I have no choice this time. I plead my case. "The numbness and tingling in my extremities are related to food. Another spinal tap will reveal nothing."

"I have to rule out the possibility of MS," he explains.

"How do you intend to treat me if I have MS?"

"There is no treatment for MS at the beginning stages," he says.

"Why is it important to rule out MS, if there's no treatment?"

"If you don't consent to the spinal tap, the gastroenterology team will not treat you." What choice do I have? My hands are tied.

The gastroenterology team have just topped off my day by announcing that the barium enema was negative.

The pen scribbles my pent up thoughts. Don, nothing has improved since you left. I've given up. Nothing but negative tests. Why am I being punished? The new year hasn't brought any solutions. I've lost more weight and that really worries me. I'm scared to step on the scale. My feistiness and sense of humor are quickly disappearing. I have no more hope. I never thought Heather Millar would give up, but she has.

As I read over the letter, I realize that I can't send it to Don. I want to share my thoughts and feelings with him, but the letter is too depressing. I tuck it away in the drawer.

Later, I lie on the testing table, enjoying the warmth from the jelly the ultrasound tech has placed on my stomach. Each day my body seems to become more sensitive to the cold. Is this due to my continuing weight loss? The tech is focusing on a particularly tender area under my ribs, the area where I experience the most pain. I wince when she presses down. She calls the radiologist over to look at the monitor. What do they see? Nothing that they'll reveal to me.

Four o'clock. The flu-like feeling is back. I feel sluggish, cold, and overwhelmingly sick. My hip joints hurt. My records reveal that exactly eight hours have passed since I ate my morning egg.

## January 21

My third spinal tap is scheduled for today. Why was my spinal fluid not tested for MS previously? The symptoms haven't changed from those I first experienced in Memphis. This test is really distressing. Repeating it for the third time is poor planning.

What to do with my free hour before the test. A walk outside the hospital, without the companionship of the IV pole and a wheelchair, will be a treat. In my weakened condition, I can't be too adventurous, but I can walk on my own. The air smells fresh and sweet, a welcome contrast to the stagnant hospital air always reeking of disinfectant. I wish I could run away from the hospital, from life. I know I'm sick. Why are all the tests negative? I don't understand.

I head toward a bookstore, a place that reminds me of standing in a long line to buy textbooks, during the first weeks of classes. My days as a student defined by friends, parties, and classes. I didn't think so then, but life as a student was so simple. Can I find solutions here to this problem which has haunted me for months? As I stand in the medical section reviewing the different books, the pervasive feeling of weakness slowly breaks into my consciousness. I must return to the hospital.

Do I have enough strength to return to the ward? The road inclines slightly for almost a block. Although the slope is minimal, I don't have enough reserves to meet the challenge and I search for an easier route, finally making my way back.

The aching in my hips is more pronounced today than during the previous spinal taps. The first stab of freezing is unusually painful, and the medication stings as it enters my flesh. The spinal needle burns as it pierces my back. I shouldn't feel a burning sensation.

"I can feel the needle burning," I say in a distressed voice. Doctor N3 stops, injects more freezing, and stabs me a second time. The needle still burns when he injects it. Something isn't right.

# The Toxic Labyrinth

"Stop!"

He injects more freezing. How much more do I have to endure until he gets the procedure right? I know this test will prove nothing.

After thirty minutes and three unsuccessful attempts, I refuse to continue. My knuckles, white and covered with my tears, are glued to the bed rail. Doctor N3 apologizes. He'll return later in the afternoon to try again. I know he has no choice. The doctor who supervises him is anxious for the results. He has shown the most compassion of any of the doctors I've seen. Sitting at my bedside, he offers soothing words of encouragement and seems truly sorry he has to perform the test. Upset and oblivious to his words, I just want him to leave.

Did my children perceive me as an insensitive, distant figure who came into their lives to inflict pain, or as a caring mother figure who made their life a little easier? The institutional atmosphere seems, at times, to rob us of our humanity.

Alone, I lie on my bed looking at the ceiling, the pain rippling up my back. I've been subjected to testing for months without the comfort of a diagnosis. I cry uncontrollably, not caring who hears. I want to go home. I shiver, a reminder that the flu-like signs are back.

The nurse has come into my room to check on me.

"Do you need anything?" she asks.

"No, I'm fine."

She has seen my tears and has returned with some pain medication. I smile at her thoughtfulness, holding the pills in my hand until she leaves. No unnecessary medication for me. I put the pills into the drawer of my bedside table.

Mom has caught the last of my tears and we discuss the morning's horrors. She will stay and act as my buffer; there will be no more testing today.

The neurology team is lined up at the foot of my bed, soldiers ready to carry out orders. With Mom by my side, I have the strength to resist their advances. The next spinal tap will have to wait until the end of the weekend. No more stabs into my flesh for now. The head doctor glances at Mom's resolute face, decides not to push the issue, and leaves.

**January 22**

Condition unchanged. My body is sluggish and the constant joint pains make walking difficult. I'm eating small meals to maintain my nutrition, while keeping my symptoms to a minimum. The daily food record clearly demonstrates a relationship between eating and the symptoms, which is obvious to anyone reads my notes. Why do the tests not confirm my theory of Crohn's disease?

I've finally eliminated all the barium absorbed during the enema. I can see clots of blood throughout my stool, yet no one is interested in my findings, even though my condition improved immediately, once the barium left my body.

**January 24**

The endoscopy, a procedure to reveal any abnormalities from the upper part of the throat to the stomach, requires an IV. As the IV nurse searches my pale hands for a suitable vein, she comments that my veins are not in good shape. Her remark strikes an ominous chord.

Another sigmoidoscopy has been scheduled, in addition to the endoscopy. These tests still avoid the only part of my body I feel is relevant to my problem, the small intestine, the area where Crohn's disease was first diagnosed. But the sigmoidoscopy may produce some clues.

The porters move a steady stream of patients through the doors of the examination room. So many people have bowel problems, yet no one feels comfortable discussing this condition, and I can relate. Despite the fact I've had pains and nausea for years, I don't discuss my bowel habits. Is there a delicate way to discuss the bowel. I certainly wouldn't converse about my bowel at a party, but a herniated disc, a sprained ankle, or even a kidney stone are acceptable conditions.

The long, thick, black scope lies curled on the tray, a snake-like instrument waiting to slither down my throat. The medicine had better work. I want no memory of this procedure.

I chat with the nurse as she explains the procedure. First she will spray my throat with a freezing agent. I should hold my breath while she sprays, because the spray is very uncomfortable if it enters the lungs. When she sprays, my throat burns and my chest tightens. My throat is becoming numb, and I'm losing the ability to swallow. One look at me tells her what I'm experiencing. Assuring me that I won't choke, she sprays my throat again. Now I can't swallow at all. She injects a syringe full of clear fluid into my IV. Is it the right drug and the right amount? A plastic mouth guard so I won't bite the scope...

Both tests are over. I'm relaxed. Just take me back to my room so I can sleep.

Doctor N3 is waiting to perform the return engagement of the spinal tap. More sedation. Who cares what they do to me? It's a great day.

**January 25**

The neurology team is gathered around my bed for a pending announcement. The head doctor lowers his voice, sucks in his breath, looks me directly in the eyes, and proclaims the verdict. I don't have MS. What a surprise!! Their in-depth testing has revealed nothing. He pronounces the standard diagnosis, anxiety attacks.

ANXIETY ATTACKS!! Is this the best they can do? I confront the head doctor. "What about the abnormal count of white cells in my spinal fluid? What about the weakness you detected on my left side the last time I was in hospital? I can't make up those results."

He casually replies that both the weakness and the white blood cells have disappeared. With all my strength, I push myself to the edge of the bed and in a tone laced with disbelief, I voice my opinion. "I have traveled through Thailand, ridden an elephant in the hills by the Cambodian border, and worked in pediatric hospitals in some of the most dangerous urban areas in the United States. I'm not an anxious person. The diagnosis doesn't fit my personality."

He shrugs his shoulders, "Anxiety can affect anyone, anytime, anywhere," and suggests treatment with an anti-depressant medication.

Disgusted, I look at them and state emphatically, "No, I refuse to take anti-depressants."

I'm furious. All these tests and still no answers. Why can't they piece this thing together? I start to cry out of anger and frustration, but quickly catch myself. Seeing me cry will only confirm their diagnosis.

The morning has gone from bad to worse. The endoscopy, ultrasound, and sigmoidoscopy were all negative. What's my next step?

"Mom, they keep saying that I'm anxious and depressed."

"We both know that you are neither. Be patient. We have to keep gathering more information to find the answer. I still think we will find your condition is related to food in some way."

Doctor G2 has scheduled one more test for tomorrow, a CT scan of my abdomen. I can have the test as an outpatient, so I'm going home. There's no sense in adding the expense of another night's hospitalization to my mounting medical costs.

No one believes I'm sick. I've been discharged without a reasonable diagnosis. At least I feel a little better and can eat some solid food.

# The Toxic Labyrinth

**January 26**

In preparation for the scan, I've followed the instructions and managed to drink the contrast media, more radio active dye for my body. The flu-like feeling has returned this morning, clouding my vision, making the dull-colored walls of the waiting room appear fuzzy. How long can I sit upright? Is there no place to lie down?

Another IV! They didn't explain this procedure required an IV. If I had known, I wouldn't have let them remove the IV catheter from my hand before I was discharged. It could have been capped for use, one last time. In anger and frustration, I thrust my arm out to the nurse who is holding the tourniquet.

The tech hands me another pint of contrast to drink. How can I manage to drink more of this metal tasting liquid? She tells me to hurry. There are people lined up waiting for testing. The last test, this will be the last test. I will myself to make it through the next hour. Containing my urge to vomit, I finish the remaining liquid.

Contrast dye will also be administered though an IV. I explain to the tech my reaction to the type of contrast dye used in Memphis. She assures me I shouldn't have any problem. Before she leaves the room, she connects the IV and starts the solution infusing.

The sticky solution is spraying me in the face! I turn away to avoid getting any more in my eyes. Moving my arms disconnects the IV and contaminates the tubing. The solution has gone everywhere, except into the vein. IV solution covers my face, and blood is spurting from the IV site. I don't care to see what will happen next and turn away from the whole scene. Tears slide silently down my cheeks making rivulets through the dye. I shudder and wonder how much more of this I can take.

The dye infuses, bringing with it the sickening warmth. The taste of metal is strong and increases my nausea. Shifting on the table, I gasp for breath. Over the loud-speaker from inside her booth, the tech commands me to remain still.

"I feel sick!" I shout.

"The test won't last much longer."

It's the last test, and I have to hang on no matter how sick I feel.

Home, at last, I lie on the sofa huddled under the blankets to ward off the cold that persists, regardless of the room temperature. My head hurts and my lower legs are aching and cold. The clock registers exactly eight hours from the time I ingested the contrast media.

A short clear period to do something other than languish inside the apartment. The mailbox is only half a block away, but it may as well be three miles. I push myself forward, gathering the strength to reach my destination. The red metal box seems to ridicule my determined effort to lift my arms and place the letter in the slot.

## January 28

Connie smokes a cigarette while we visit at the restaurant. How unusual, I can't stand the smell of the smoke, and my chest feels tight. The room is reeling; the claustrophobia is overwhelming. Can the cigarette smoke be causing these symptoms? I've spent many social hours in smoky bars with no adverse effects.

My lungs suck in the outside air, and slowly I start to recover. I'll remember the effects of the smoke. Why did it trigger my symptoms?

It's not so painfully difficult to walk today. Symptoms plague me during the day, but only during the usual times of early morning and evening. I ignore the discomfort and carry on.

Val and Eric are having a birthday party for me. I've gone on clear fluids again to clear my symptoms, so it's difficult watching everyone eat and drink. I'll try to be spirited and vivacious. At least I'm at a party and not in the hospital. Have I turned the corner?

**CHAPTER 6**

# DARK PASSAGE

I touch the cold, hard walls of the passage. The barrier stands unyielding and surrenders no clues.

# The Toxic Labyrinth

## February 1

Today is my thirty-first birthday. The usual all night celebration has been replaced by a quiet evening with Mom at a play, and a dozen long stem red roses from Don. I miss him so much and count the days until he is with me again. Knowing he is standing by me through this keeps me going.

Four months, I've been ill for a third of a year. It's hard to believe what has happened to me, the hospitals, the doctors. But I'm feeling somewhat better today, and maybe good health will be my birthday present.

## February 2

A hair cut and pampering at the salon, projects to uplift my spirits, are my goals for the afternoon. The steep hill rising like a monument to my weakened body makes the unmanageable incline a week ago seem insignificant. But I'm ready for new challenges, and I must conquer this barrier that stands between home and the salon.

I'm half way to the top, managing the ascent with little objection from my body. I cheer silently as I reach the pinnacle. I *will* make myself well. I *am* determined.

Not only a haircut, but a manicure and pink nails to help me celebrate my freedom from the hospital. In the back room the beautician begins to work her magic. What's she saying to me? Her words are jumbled like pieces of a jigsaw puzzle laying in a pile. I can't assemble them to make any sense. The hand she's working on appears hazy, as if a semi-transparent film has been placed over my eyes. The smell of the manicuring products is nauseating. The room is starting to revolve. One more nail, just one more nail.

"Can I dry my nails outside?" I ask and make a dash for the door. The fog in my brain lifts, and my surroundings cease their mad whirl. When I return to quickly pay my bill, the smells assault me once again. The excitement of being pampered has abruptly receded, replaced by a desire for the safety of home.

The smell of the rush hour exhaust is making me sick to my stomach. I can't faint, not here. Can I manage the walk home? No, I have to find a phone and call Mom to pick me up. The store is calming, a safe haven from the fumes in the street. Protected behind the closed door, I start to recover.

Mom has made a special meal of tofu lasagna with eggplant. Ravenous from my walk, I wash down the very ample portion with a large glass of orange juice.

**February 3**

My eyes snap open. What has wakened me? The crushing in my chest is the worst it's ever been. Is this what it would be like to be pinned under a building, its massive weight pushing against my chest? My feet are numb to my hips. I won't throw up; I won't give in. Will sitting up help me breathe? My hands and feet appear very heavy and far away. Are they really my hands and feet? I direct them to move, but they won't function at my command. I'll wait for the spell to pass. All my other spells have passed eventually. Hopefully this one will too.

Finally, at 6:30 a.m. I find relief and the tranquillity of sleep.

The rattling of dishes in the kitchen has awakened me. Joint pains and a sluggish feeling have replaced the oppressive sickness. My mind is racing as it tries to make sense of my early morning episode. I'd been feeling so much better. Why does the answer keep eluding me?

Eating my lunch of leftovers from the night before, I think about Carol, a close friend from high school days. Carol understands me, the real me, the person I used to be. Getting out of the apartment and visiting with her will be a wonderful treat.

## The Toxic Labyrinth

The doorbell summons me to action. Trying to move quickly, I walk to the top of the stairs, the flu-like feeling slowly seeping into my limbs. If I pretend nothing is wrong, Carol won't know how sick I really am. It's important for me to put on a happy face and keep going. Life is for living. I've endured stomach aches since I was in high school, and had I stayed home every time I felt unwell, I would never have gone anywhere. I've worked, partied, and carried on a normal life despite the chronic pain. My motto is to make the best of what I have, but lately I'm finding it harder to live by this. Carol is standing at the bottom of the stairs. Can I make it down? I will my legs to make the descent.

The street is littered with bits and pieces of my energy, squandered during the walk to the restaurant. I arrive depleted, with little stamina remaining to talk, much less to make witty, interesting conversation. As I try to focus on what Carol is saying, the words flow across my brain, some making sense while others are lost in transit.

Back home, relieved I don't have to make an effort at being sociable, I collapse into bed and succumb to the controlling exhaustion.

### February 4

All my symptoms are back with a vengeance. From time to time, the waves of sickness wash away, offering a brief remission in the form of fitful and intermittent sleep. Finally, I give up on sleep and prop myself up on the pillow. Will I ever get well? In the morning, I'll call Doctor G2.

Fighting back the nausea, I explain my situation. Doctor G2 listens and replies, "It sounds to me like you are having panic attacks, again." He suggests I follow the recommendation of the neurology team and take some anti-depressant medication. As far as he's concerned, the bowel symptoms I'm having are in my head.

However, if clear fluids make me feel better, I can go back on that regimen.

I hang up the phone, feelings of anger and helplessness jostling for my attention. This condition is not the same as living with chronic stomach pain. Although that pain was uncomfortable, I had adjusted my life around it. This existence on clear fluids is precarious, a threat to my survival. I have to eat. The constant weight loss concerns me. How can I improve my nutrition and stabilize my weight loss when I can't eat normally? I have to find someone who'll listen, someone who can offer a solution. Panic attacks and anxiety are not credible diagnoses. I know my body is physically ill. Why do the tests not show what my body is clearly signaling?

Mom and I discuss the next step. I'll make an appointment to see Doctor I1, the internist who saw me in emergency when I first arrived home from Memphis in December. He appeared to believe me.

**February 6**

Mom refuses to give up, suggesting again that I may have a food allergy. I have focused on the fact that my condition could be connected to Crohn's disease and put aside the allergy theory. She helps me down the stairs to her office. Together we sign on to a health data base on Internet. As we pull up articles on food allergy and start to read, the evidence of the relationship between my symptoms and allergies becomes clearer. The riddle is beginning to make sense. I'm eating bland food to rest my irritated bowel, but most of these bland foods: eggs, tofu (soy), bread (wheat) and pasta (wheat) are the worst offenders for people with food allergies. Thankfully I had eliminated alcohol when I started the fungal medication, and coffee after my hospitalization in December.

What had I eaten before the onset of my last symptoms? I couldn't have eaten a worse meal, every food that is high on the allergy scale: pasta, orange juice, eggplant, tomatoes, and soy. Have we found the reason for the constant assaults on my body? By using my daily records and reaching back into my memory, we assemble some more pieces of the puzzle. Don's passion for cooking pasta. Crawfish season in New Orleans. Meals of crackers and prepared meats with Daryl. The pasta on Bowen Island. Lobster and pasta during the Christmas holidays. The list goes on and on.

I think back to my last few days in the hospital. Because my tests had shown a prolonged bleeding time, an indication of vitamin K deficiency, I had added broccoli to my diet rather than endure the vitamin injections. Broccoli is a high fiber food. If I have Crohn's disease, I shouldn't be able to tolerate broccoli. The allergy theory is starting to make sense.

**February 7**

I close my eyes and wait for the 2 a.m. symptoms to pass, vivid reminders of the pasta and tomatoes I ate for dinner.

Although my symptoms are the worst in the very early morning hours, my regular waking time is usually the best period of my day. However, this morning my symptoms have escalated, a turn of events that convinces me I have to make an appointment with an allergist.

What will the allergist, Doctor Al, say? I fill out the comprehensive, two page form, noting all the symptoms which have tormented me for months are listed on the questionnaire. Maybe this doctor can offer the solution I so desperately need.

I relate my story and hand the doctor my weighty file. He quickly looks through it. Without examining me, he states that I have severe allergies, and recommends I drink a supplement he has developed. After ten days, I can start adding foods to my diet. After showing me a sample, he gives me an instruction sheet and a list of stores where I can purchase the supplement. Some of his comments make sense, but I am suspicious of taking anything which is not proven. So many of my problems have resulted from ingesting liquids and pills. I'll have to look elsewhere for advice.

I always start to feel worse after I'm out of bed and moving around. The trip to the doctor's office has triggered my symptoms. When I try to close my hands, they fail to grasp my bag, and so I tuck it under my arm.

Even my space on the sofa is no refuge today. My face is going numb, and I can't feel my eyes when they blink. Nausea envelops me. Why? I've only had water to drink today.

I call frantically, "Mom, help me to the bathroom!"

I begin to retch uncontrollably. I can't feel my face. My throat is swelling shut. I try to convey my panic to Mom. Violent pains stabbing at my stomach, burning in the back of my neck, and crushing chest pain deplete what little energy I have. Holding on to the sides of the toilet, I retch while Mom rubs my back and wipes my face with a cool, damp cloth. Dying would be preferable to this.

What medication did I give my children when they had violent, allergic reactions to their blood transfusions? Antihistamine. Maybe that will help calm my body. I swallow the medication and fight the nausea to keep it down. Soon the burning in my eyes and the numbness in my face subside.

Another hour has passed. The strength is returning to my hands and the pressure inside my face has cleared. I can function almost normally. Only a slight shortness of breath remains. I'm excited. Have we found the answer? When my body settles down completely, I can start eating again. I know the direction to go.

**February 8**

A night of sleep, without numbness or nausea. My breakfast is a drink of water. The slight symptoms, once I am up and moving about, remind me of yesterday's horror; and I decide to take an antihistamine, a precaution against the swelling in the roof of my mouth, the shortness of breath, and the tingling in my legs.

I love children. Baby-sitting Brenda for Connie is my treat for today. Brenda sits and plays quietly with her toys or I hold her on my lap, while we watch cartoon videos and laugh at the colorful images of Aladdin and the Genie.

In the early evening, Mom returns from her business trip to Victoria and hands me a small stone used as a talisman by the First Nations people. They believe the medicine stone has the power to heal the person who carries it.

"May the stone bring you good health. It's important to search for answers wherever we can find them, to use whatever we can to make you well." She hugs me and places the stone in my hand.

The numbness has returned to my face and the freezing cold to my hands and feet. I swallow more antihistamine. I haven't had anything to eat today, so my symptoms must be from the wheat I've eaten in the last week. I lie in bed, my feet like ice inside the heavy socks, my chest pulling with each breath. In spite of these symptoms, tonight I'm less afraid, knowing I have a path to follow.

## February 9

The clock shows just after midnight. What has wakened me? Where am I? I grab the phone. I need to call someone, but who do I call? My arms are numb. My hands are numb. I'm having difficulty swallowing. I gasp for breath and try to sit up. The phone is still in my hand. The confusion clears, and I realize I'm home. I dial Mom's bedroom phone.

"Mom, I can't breathe. My throat is closing." I pick up my inhaler and take a long breath. The bank of fog is quickly forming. "Hospital. I have to go to the hospital."

I feel as if hands are closing slowly, tightly around my throat as the car speeds faster through the snow and sleet. Mom is calling ahead on the cellular phone to alert the emergency room. ". . . possible this is anaphylactic shock." I have not been to this hospital before. My condition and the bad weather have made its proximity the only suitable choice.

I'm being grilled about my medical history and I don't want to recount my complicated history once more. I just want them to stop the gasping and retching, to let me see the doctor. A cardiac monitor is attached to my chest. My breathing is starting to ease and the tightness around my throat is loosening. The shaking begins, a welcome change in my body, because it heralds the departure of the worst symptoms.

Doctor ER3 examines me and commences his history. But wait. I've mentioned my treatment at another hospital just last month. Cutting me off mid story, he takes another look at the file I have given him with all my test results, the file that creates a medical image by virtue of its size.

"Nothing is physically wrong with you. I would advise psychiatric follow up." He has reinforced the diagnosis of the neurologists by looking at my throat.

I'm sick, but more than that, I am angry. Shaking, my numb fingers fumble as I wrestle with the ties on the hospital gown. I'll never come back. How can a health care professional have treated me so callously? Mom says information gives people power. Some day I'll have information these people don't have. I will get well, if only to prove to them I'm not crazy. Mustering energy from unknown reserves, I hold my head high and walk out the front door.

Another fruitless trip with no reasonable solutions. I have disturbed my family in the middle of the night for nothing. This unrelenting illness is making me tired, is making my family tired. Are allergies the whole answer? I haven't eaten today, yet my symptoms still persist.

# The Toxic Labyrinth

For the remainder of the night my retching and vomiting continue. The pain in my chest is constant. Oh, God how I miss Don. I'm trying to make myself well, and nothing is working.

Mid afternoon and I've become impatient, tired of the numbness, tingling, and nausea. The wheat from the pasta that I've eaten must be lodged in my bowel, causing this prolonged set of symptoms. While it remains in my body, I know it will make me ill. A children's laxative, the same brand and dosage I took in the hospital, should clear my system. What made me feet better in the hospital should work at home.

The laxative is beginning to take effect. Am I going to faint? My body is shaky and weak, my legs cold and numb. Perspiration runs down my forehead as the nausea and retching intensify.

After a while, I feel the improvement: warm hands and feet, no weakness, numbness, or shortness of breath. The feeling of agitation has subsided. Plenty of chicken soup, water, and apple juice should keep me from dehydrating. If I begin a new regimen and stop eating all those bland foods that were making me sick, I should see some progress.

Before going to bed, I brush my teeth and my chest starts to burn. Am I reacting to the toothpaste? Impossible, since I've always used this brand. The burning is just a coincidence.

**February 10**

It's 5 a.m. and I'm retching. The burning in the back of my neck has returned, and my hip joints are on fire. How can I start my new diet today if these symptoms persist?

By 9 a.m. I'm watching the sail boats bob in their moorings in the marina below while I cautiously take inventory of my body for trouble spots. All is calm. I walk downstairs to Mom's office and announce my good fortune.

My sense of well-being is fleeting. The nausea and shortness of breath have crept silently back, and the pain across the back of my neck comes in waves. Thinking the attendant weakness results from a lack of sugar, I push myself toward the kitchen, supporting my body on pieces of furniture as I go. With the sugar against my cheek, I lie down to watch TV until it's time to leave for my appointment with Doctor Il.

It's no longer possible to swallow apple juice or water. The light is breaking into black, opaque shards. Suddenly, I can see nothing, nothing but black.

"Mom, I have to go to the hospital, *now*." I can't wait another three hours for my appointment. I have to see the doctor immediately. "Help me take a bath before we go."

Mom is incredulous. "How can you think about taking a bath when you can barely stand?"

I have this premonition that I won't return home for many days and I desperately want to bathe before leaving. Walking toward the bathroom, I collapse in the hallway when the blackness overtakes me once more. Mom's words are muffled: ". . . to the hospital in my car?" I try to answer. Silence. Our fear reverberates from the walls as Mom calls the ambulance.

The paramedics have arrived; their words are indistinguishable from Mom's. Familiar sounds reach my semi-consciousness: the metal scrape of the portable stretcher, the hiss of air from the blood pressure cuff. Even though I'm in a state of collapse, my vital signs indicate I'm well enough to manage the trip to the hospital where Doctor Il practices.

As I fade in and out of consciousness, the claustrophobic, metal coffin announces my passage through streets choked with noon-hour traffic. I hold the oxygen mask to my face, the smell of the plastic permeating my lungs. I reach into my back pocket and clutch the medicine stone in the palm of my hand, praying to whatever gods are inside for their healing powers.

# The Toxic Labyrinth

More questions from the ambulance attendant, so I try to focus, but I can't follow her questioning. The feeling I had experienced in Memphis is back. I can hear and see, but no longer speak. My hands resist my control; fingers with no sensation move in front of my face. I'm losing my grip on the medicine stone. A black veil slides across my vision. Thoughts, muddled and chaotic, signal that I'm slipping into shock! "More oxygen." I grab the mask, while the attendant tilts the head of my stretcher towards the floor, forcing the blood into my head.

My vision is clearing. I can move my hands a little. "Keep tilting the stretcher," I demand. "How much farther to the hospital?" I hold on to the stone and pray.

The energy of the emergency room swirls through my fog. Numerous nurses come and go, attending to their duties in my cubicle. Murmurs from the staff conversing about my case drift through the curtain. The IV nurse sounds doubtful about being able to hit a vein in my hand. An arm stretches across the sheet. Whose arm is so blue? The nurse sets the IV solution to drip as fast as it will go. I breathe more oxygen. I want Mom beside me, but she's not allowed into the emergency room. There is no more pain. Am I going to die alone? Is this what dying is like, no flurry just calm?

Mom stands by the bed and takes my hand. The dream-like state is gone, and I can concentrate more easily. My body, greedy for the saline solution, has rapidly sucked the contents of the IV bag into my tissues. The medicine stone presses against my palm, reminding me that I have succeeded in holding it throughout the ordeal.

Doctor I1 is sympathetic and gives the impression he believes me. Although my case is complex, one that he thinks is beyond his scope, he will decide on the best route for me to take.

This is my sixth hospital admission. Not only is my roster of medical professionals growing daily, but tests are constantly repeated when a new expert comes into the picture. What I had thought was a two-week problem has evolved into an ongoing mysterious illness no one seems to fathom. The only bright spot is that I now qualify for coverage under the Canadian health care system.

I always try to be personable no matter how badly I'm feeling, readily assuming the role of the polite, cooperative patient. I don't have the energy for lengthy conversation today, and since Doctor I1 is familiar with my story, I need relate only the most recent details. After looking carefully through the information and listening to my story, he decides the root of my problem may be related to Crohn's. I groan. Not another gastroenterologist. Will this decision lead in any direction other than the two previous times I have consented to this route? I'm somewhat comforted by the fact he has promised an appointment with an allergist once I've left the hospital.

Three bags of fluid and I'm returning to my old self. Dehydration appears to be causing a problem, yet with my daily fluid intake this seems unreasonable. The nurse hangs a bag of IV fluid that appears different from the type normally given to patients suffering from dehydration. Doctor I1 must have ordered a special mixture.

I taste the dryness in my mouth, feel the fluid being sucked out of my cells. "Please, check the doctor's orders for IV fluid. I think this is the wrong preparation."

The nurse is reluctant to comply, but I'm adamant. She quickly returns with a different bag, confirming my suspicions. A quarter of the way through the new bag and my body is calm. I'll have to monitor my treatment more carefully.

My bed is next to the window for a change. Drab, gray hospital curtain has been replaced by a view of the gray sky and intermittent rain, a reflection of my mood. The oxygen mask hangs unused. Can I manage to breathe on my own? Am I going to be sick for the rest of my life? Don, why are you in Africa? I'm beyond scared. Thoughts whirl through my head, preventing any successful attempt at sleep. Hospital sounds echo from the hallway. Food trays clattering against the carts remind me I don't have to face the challenge of eating for a few days. The persistent thirst interrupts my thoughts, and I turn up my IV slightly to increase the flow.

My symptoms disappear only to reappear an hour later. Nausea and agitation wash over me in waves. In between the waves, I manage to drift off to sleep for a few minutes, wishing all the while for my thirst to diminish.

**February 11**

The sounds of conversation drift from the nursing station through the quiet of the early morning. Waves of sickness wash over me continuously. A strange, pinpoint, red rash has appeared on my lower extremities. Although the nurse glances with disinterest at it, I have accomplished my goal. The rash is documented. The patient can't imagine a rash.

Ursula is a spiritual counselor for the hospital. I've attended church very infrequently. Now I'm beginning to feel differently about the course of my life. Afraid to face each day, no longer my confident, risk taking self, I look for assistance wherever I can find it. Does she have any answers or wise words to help me through this? Any other time, I would tell her I'm not interested in listening. Today I feel the need to hear what she has to say.

Tears and words flood the room. I'm not uncomfortable with this stranger which surprises me. Do I sense that I can share my deepest, darkest thoughts with her? She says a prayer for me before she leaves, an act that gives me a small ray of hope.

Why can't I quench this insatiable thirst? As soon as I swallow water, I gag and retch. I'm thirsty, regardless of the amount of fluid the IV has pumped into my body; fluid that appears to flood my lungs and make me cough. The room has become distorted, as if I'm looking through water. I reach up and slow the rate of the IV.

They want to move me to another ward. I hardly have the strength to think about where my things are, much less pack them. I wait in the wheelchair, packed and ready for the porter who is taking an eternity. Too weak to sit erect, my head bobs against my shoulder.

The porter wheels me out into the corridor. When we round the corner, a strong smell of fresh paint invades my senses. My vision changes from clear to hazy. Nausea rises in my throat. Does the porter notice the smell?

After arriving in my new room, I'm informed that I'll be going for chest and abdominal x-rays. "Immediately?" My question is answered when the porter pulls the wheelchair up to the bedside. Do I have the physical strength? The ride to x-ray takes me once more through the paint fume miasma.

After waiting for what seemed to be an eternity, I stand in front of the machine, supported by the tech. My jelly-like legs refuse to hold me erect for the few minutes it takes to snap the film. More waiting, this time for the abdominal x-ray. Can I hold out? I lean my head against the wall for support. As I step on the stool to boost myself onto the table, I lose my balance. The tech rushes to catch me. Aware that I'm in distress, he guides me into each position. Instructions come through a haze. My whole body aches. Would I be more comfortable riding on a stretcher back to my room? I nod. Resting my head against the pillow, I close my eyes in relief.

Back in the ward, the sickness attacks with renewed vigor. I shake. My body is in pain. My legs are numb. My esophagus is burning. Periods of blackness intermingle with the more familiar sensations. Can I be fainting when I am lying down? There are no words powerful enough to describe what I am enduring at this moment.

Realizing my condition is more serious than usual, Mom calls the nurse. I try to recount my symptoms, but I'm losing my ability to concentrate. The sensations that overpowered me during the ambulance ride are returning. The room is receding. I place the oxygen mask on my face. I can't breathe in fast enough.

# The Toxic Labyrinth

The nurse wants to give me a relaxant. I refuse and ask for an antihistamine instead. As she takes the syringe and injects the antihistamine into the IV port closest to my wrist, apprehension grips me. I'm going to receive a lot of medication very quickly. The immediate sensation in my tissues is indescribable and horrendous. Is the moisture being sucked from my tissues, creating the impression that my eyes are being forced into their sockets and my esophagus thrust out of my chest?

"Mom, I need the bedpan." I have a compulsion to void, an intense action that I repeat several times with equal urgency.

Restless and agitated, I can't find a comfortable position. Oh God, I'm dying. I grab Mom's hand. I'm scared. I shouldn't feel this sick inside. What's happening to me? An older nurse enters the room. She holds my hand and speaks to me in soft, soothing tones. Calmly, she takes my vital signs and reassures me the readings are normal, actions which indicate her experience. Adjusting the oxygen mask on my face, she strokes the back of my head. My body finally begins to calm down. Although I still have an uncontrollable thirst, at least I'm not writhing on the bed. I will always remember her kindness and patience. Alone at the busiest time of the evening shift, she remained with me, assuring me the sensation would pass. This woman is unforgettable in a long list of health care workers I have met. She is a true nurse.

I lie in my bed, trying to summon my surroundings into focus. Has the antihistamine made my body better or worse? Despite the smell of the plastic mask, I breathe the oxygen, needing the sustenance it gives my body. Too weak to say much, I look over at Mom and whisper to her.

"Am I going to die? I never imagined I would be this sick. Pray for me, Mom. There's nothing left to do."

Mom squeezes my hand and reassures me again that my vital signs are fine. "I know none of us can imagine what this is like for you. You have to find the strength to keep going. If it takes everything I have, we'll find out what is wrong. You will get better."

I close my eyes. Is there a God? I grip Mom's hand tightly. I'm very afraid I'm not going to be with Mom for much longer.

My friend Bob has arrived. He's driven for forty minutes to visit me, and all I can manage is a weak hello. Looking at me, he knows I'm very ill. We've been friends for a very long time, and he's never seen me this devoid of personality or energy. He squeezes my hand and tells me that I have to get better. I'm too sick to reply.

**February 12**

Looking out at the incessant rain, the only constant in this unstable winter, I reflect on my decision to stop fighting. Black mood, black day. A conviction is building within my soul that my life is not worth living, if this what I have to endure day after day.

"Hi, Heather. Today, I can spend the whole day with you." Mom's cheery greeting breaks into my thoughts.

"Mom, I'm tired of life. Even reading passages from the Bible is not giving me strength. I'm going to give up."

"Heather, you can't give up. We'll find out what is wrong."

"No, you don't understand. No one understands what it's like to be inside my body. I'm tired of trying."

"Heather, you don't understand what the rest of us are going through. You're not the only one who is tired. We're all tired. I've come to spend the day with you. Since you've given up, I'm leaving. If you change your mind, you can phone me." Picking up her coat, she heads for the door without looking back.

Is Mom's threat serious? I've learned in the past it's not wise to call her bluff. Mom is tough and may very well leave me to fend for myself.

"Come back. I won't talk about quitting." For now anyway.

# The Toxic Labyrinth

The small, white, anti-nausea pill has been prescribed by Doctor G3, the gastroenterologist who I will be seeing on Monday. The nurse informs me this medication has been prescribed every eight hours along with ranitidine, a combination to relieve my stomach and chest symptoms. Reluctantly, I put the pill under my tongue. This is the same medication that restored the sensation to my hands in emergency. Maybe it'll be okay.

The nurse hooks the small medicine bag filled with ranitidine to my IV pole. The bag has not been premixed by the pharmacy. Did she double check the medication before she mixed it into the bag? The memory of the wrong IV solution is still fresh in my mind. The solution drips down the tubing towards my arm. My stomach is churning, and I'm nauseated. I turn on the TV for distraction, and in only a few minutes, the nausea and pain in my left arm fade into the distance. Warmth floods into my body. Closing my eyes, I drift off into uninterrupted sleep for the first time in days.

**February 13**

My roommate, critically ill after a major heart attack, cannot be disturbed. Connie and Brenda have ridden the bus for an hour to visit with me. Now that I'm able to sit up for short periods, we can visit in the lounge near my room. Just before we leave, the nurse attaches a small bag of medication to the IV.

The visit has ended much too quickly, curtailed by the onset of nausea. Back in my room, I think about cause and effect. Every time the nurse administers the ranitidine, the nausea begins. I make a mental note of this fact.

**February 14**

Doctor G3 is very brusque and matter of fact, but I've been warned about his bedside manner, and it doesn't faze me. He notes I've been observed and tested by Doctor G2, a very reputable gastroenterologist; his opinion should not be questioned. He will consult with Doctor G2 to gain more insight into my case.

Mom asks about the relationship between my symptoms and the time of day. Doctor G3 considers her question for a minute, then dismisses it as irrelevant. Eager for his opinion, I mention the information I have collected about Crohn's from the health data base. He sees no value in this activity and advises me against further research. As he strides from the room, he commands me to begin drinking fluids.

The good patient follows orders. The first few sips of apple juice make my esophagus burn immediately. The homemade chicken soup creates no burning, just slight nausea.

Beginning with a number of gastrointestinal investigations, the battery of testing is ramping up again. Even though I have begged Doctor G3 to wait as long as possible, at least until I feel a little better, he's given me just two days grace.

Mom has brought Valentine's Day flowers from Don. He always makes arrangements for wonderful bouquets to be delivered weekly when he is in Nigeria. Since this is a special occasion, I have an extra floral treat. The teddy bear with his arms wrapped around the heart-shaped vase sits on the bedside table, reminding me that Don will be home in three days. I miss him, but I dread having to conduct our life from a hospital room.

**February 15**

Mardi Gras. I look out the window. Sadness overcomes me. In four years, I have not missed a Mardi Gras celebration in New Orleans. Lisa, Karen, and Paulette will be partying without me. The streets of the city will be filled with people catching the green, gold, and purple beads and eating King Cake.

# The Toxic Labyrinth

No reaction when I drink the water. Am I improving? My nutrition has really suffered in the last month. As if to second my thoughts, the bottle of vitamins beckons me from my bedside table. Immediately after swallowing a pill, a violent wave of nausea washes over me, and I start to retch.

## February 16

Tonight I have started taking the ranitidine orally rather than by IV, only to experience the same pressure rising in my esophagus. Am I allergic to this medication? I've read that asthmatics don't tolerate it well.

No eating after midnight, because special blood work has been ordered for the morning. This restriction presents no problem for me. I'm constantly nauseated and must force myself to eat.

## February 17

Little pangs of hunger growl insistently in the quiet of the room. The pill I have just taken seems have caused my hunger. A fine time for this to happen. No real appetite in the last week, and suddenly, the night I'm denied food, my body craves it. I'll close my eyes and think of other things. It's no more than a few minutes after midnight. What if I nibble on one rice cake? As long as the nurse doesn't catch me, no one will know. Hunger wins, and I wolf down the rice cake.

By 2:30 a.m. the intermittent pain in my left arm, my constant companion since Memphis which has receded in the last week, returns, adding to my discomfort. My body functions alternate between pangs of hunger and the unbearable pain in my left arm. Anticipating a long night, I pace back and forth in my room. Hunger engulfs my thoughts, and my arm aches, making sleep impossible. I increase my pacing. Strangely enough, in spite of the hunger and the pain in my arm, I don't remember feeling this well in a long time.

I'm overjoyed to see the lab tech. No sooner does the needle leave my arm, than Mom's specially prepared cold chicken and rice soup slides down my throat. I can't wait to finish the last spoonful, so I can refill the bowl; hunger is wonderful.

The dietitian and I have discussed my suspicions about allergies and she has left materials to assist me. I pore over the information. The list of problematic foods confirms my findings from Internet. If I'm going to get off this merry-go-round, I have to know more about allergies and devise a plan. The retching and vomiting disturb my reading. My watch indicates barely an hour has passed since I gave the vitamin pills one more try. What could possibly be the problem with them?

As I'm heaving into the basin, the nurse appears with instructions for the pint of contrast dye I have to drink for the abdominal CT scan. I look at the container, consider her request, and instruct her to leave the cup by the bedside. I'll attempt this task when I'm feeling better. I shake my head as she leaves. How can I drink this nasty liquid while I'm throwing up?

**February 18**

My stomach has settled after taking some anti-nausea medication, but I have quietly dumped the antacid into the sink, the less medication the better. The contrast dye awaiting my attention dredges up graphic memories of my last abdominal CT scan. It wasn't that long ago I was sprayed in the face with the contrast. But maybe Doctor G3 is correct to reorder this test. He mentioned the results from my previous abdominal CT scan revealed an unexplained thickening in my bowel. Why did no one mentioned this fact to me? Do I have both allergies and Crohn's?

I pick up the cup of fluid and take a sip. The metal taste overpowers the apple juice in the mixture. It takes ninety minutes and a lot of resolve, before the last drops leave the bottom of the cup.

# The Toxic Labyrinth

The burning in my gut forces me awake. My insides are on fire, and I start to retch. Another long night of sickness reaches out before me.

Exhausted from a night of intermittent sleep, I need some prodding from the nurse to awaken. Nausea rises in my throat as soon as I climb into the wheelchair.

The procedure nurse puts me on the stretcher to start a new IV. How many times have I been poked for blood tests or IVs? I'm cold. I want to throw up, but I have to concentrate on lying still so she can start the IV. The nurse can tell by my face that I'm ill. When she finishes taping the catheter into place, she quietly tells me to rest on the stretcher. I thank her and lie back, trying not to think about the pint of metal tasting fluid I have to choke back before my test.

I shake with chills. The waves of sickness ebb and flow, while I attempt to swallow the fluid. The bottle of IV contrast is ready. Hopefully, I'll be fine. This solution has not made me as ill as others. When I explain to the tech that I don't do very well with dye, he promises to remain with me for most of the procedure. I recognize the sickening warmth from the contrast fluid as it enters my circulation, immediately affecting my whole body. Gasping for air, I fight the sensation of claustrophobia. I'm restless and barely able to remain still.

Back in my room, I make light conversation with Mom while I wait for Don, who will arrive in a couple of hours. Unexpectedly, my bedside curtains part. Don engulfs me in his arms, the smell of Africa and his warmth accentuating his presence. Even though I'm ill, everything looks brighter now that he's back. Although he's been awake for twenty-four hours, Don quietly listens to the words that tumble out. I rush to tell him everything that has happened: the doctors that don't hear what I have to say, the recurring symptoms. Giving me a sympathetic hug, he agrees it is difficult to get anyone to recognize the role food is playing in this mysterious illness.

The flu-like symptoms have appeared six hours after drinking the contrast dye. Waves of nausea cause me to gag. The pain at the back of my neck imitates knives constantly stabbing. My right flank aches. To assure that I don't have even one hour free from medication of some kind, the nurse has brought a laxative in preparation for the gastric emptying study on Monday.

At least one bright spot looms on the horizon, a day pass for tomorrow.

**February 19**

Don has arrived to take me out for the day pass. Before leaving for my special day, I swallow another laxative and a ranitidine. Despite some shortness of breath, I want to forget about my problems.

Mom has prepared a special dinner, a family meal in my honor. It conforms to the restrictions of the allergy free diet. I eat a huge plateful of lamb, sweet potatoes, carrots, and pears. What a treat to be free from nausea for even a little while.

The day has passed quickly and it's time to return to the hospital. When my children with cancer were allowed to go out for the day, they would be so excited the night before, just as I was. I would always see tears and sad, little faces in the evening when they had to leave their families. Now I'm being left behind at the hospital. Don hugs me good bye and wipes away my tears. He reminds me that tomorrow we have another day together.

The cycle of medication begins once more, laxative followed by ranitidine.

The burning in the back of my neck is so severe I can't concentrate on the TV. All my symptoms are back. I lie back waiting for the waves of sickness to go away.

# The Toxic Labyrinth

## February 20

I'm fainting. How can I faint in my sleep? I push the call bell. The responding nurse takes my vital signs and remarks that my blood pressure is a very low, 80/40. Why is my blood pressure so low at certain times? I should call if I feel any worse. Any worse?? I'm the definition of worse.

The morning light makes patterns on the bedcovers. Another day without rain, but I won't be able to enjoy it. I'm too sick to leave the hospital. Numbness and tingling in my legs and the flu-like symptoms rack my body.

Don doesn't ask any questions. He knows what has happened by the tears streaming down my face. So much of what my cancer children went through is becoming my reality. How many times did I hold and comfort them when they were too sick to go out on a scheduled pass? Before this, I could only imagine their disappointment.

## February 21

The technician plans to observe the food as it travels through my stomach and record any problems with the digestive process. I managed to postpone the study once before when I refused to eat bread, the food commonly used for this test, because of my suspicions about allergies. Now I have special permission to eat an egg instead. As usual, no one is listening to my request for no dye. The egg will be treated with radioactive dye.

The tech is trying to make the test as easy as possible. With good intentions, he blackens the egg with pepper to make it taste more palatable. Unfortunately, he doesn't know anything about stomach problems. The last thing I want on my food is pepper.

My stomach is on fire, and I can't drink anything for two hours. In spite of this raging inferno, the test is pleasantly easy.

Don and I make the best of our time together, even though we are confined to my hospital room. Sometimes we lie on the bed watching TV. Often he reads aloud to distract me, especially when the symptoms make it difficult for me to concentrate on anything except the rhythm of his voice. He brings board games for us to play, and although he dislikes them, he participates because I enjoy this diversion.

Tonight my attention strays from the game, when an intense wave of sickness spreads through my body. My throat is swelling, and the aching joints and the flu-like feeling are settling in. A burning sensation spreads over my back, face, and hands. When I start to retch, Don calls the nurse. She takes my temperature and finds that I have a fever. Six hours have passed since I ingested the radioactive egg.

My body has settled for the moment, and the nurse is right on cue with the next hurdle, a twelve-cup jug of solution, the first of four I have to consume for tomorrow's test. I can't imagine drinking bottles of this laxative fluid before morning. Taking the first drink, I pronounce it to be nasty stuff. Don and I make jokes. How else can we cope with the situation? I tell him that this turn of events terminates our visit unless we continue our game in the bathroom.

Finally, the test *I* have wanted, a look at my small intestine, is going to be a reality. Doctor G3 should have a good look tomorrow. There is absolutely nothing left inside me. Although I'm not looking forward to the actual test, I'm definitely interested in knowing the results.

**February 22**

No interruptions last night, and I have awakened rested. Lying on my stretcher until they are ready for me, I listen to the crying sounds emanating from the testing room; the patient ahead of me is putting a voice to pain.

# The Toxic Labyrinth

I idly chat with the doctor as he prepares for the test. The nurse hands him a syringe filled with clear liquid. He plunges the shaft of the needle into my arm, piercing the flesh inside my elbow. The room has an artificial look, like a stage set observed from a distance. All my cares have vanished. The faint discomfort is so far away it must belong to someone else.

Floating on the edge of consciousness, I look over at Doctor G3 who is jotting down notes. I want to clear my mind, to ask questions, but my mind cooperates in a rather limited way. I manage one question. Could he see into the right place in my small intestine? The procedure is tricky, and I hope his efforts have not been in vain. With a yes, he puts my mind at ease. If he could see into my small intestine, we must have an answer.

Temperature normal for the first time since Memphis, my day is progressing nicely. I have eaten a huge meal of foods low on the allergy scale. If I'm going to get better, I must have patience.

Six hours after my test and I can feel my chest getting tighter. Someday I will learn why I seem to be allergic to the dyes and medicines.

**February 23**

Doctor G3 has insisted on one more test, a small bowel enema. As usual, no one has prepared me. The assumption is, incorrectly, that a nurse should know what is in store. Of all the tests, this one has to tie for first place with the barium enema for the most torturous and invasive test. I truly believe these two procedures could be used to pry information from military prisoners.

I have climbed on a stretcher to wait while the procedure nurse collects her supplies. Returning to the room, she explains the first step which involves sliding a tube up my nose and down into my stomach. I cringe at the thought of this procedure, one I had acquired an intimate knowledge of in nursing school. To improve our competence in nasogastric insertion, we had the unforgettable experience of using each other as guinea pigs. A repeat performance isn't something I desire.

As the nurse lays out the tube, my eyes widen with dismay. She can't be serious. This tube, the diameter of a garden hose, is going up my nose? In nursing school we had used pediatric tubes, and that was painful enough. I grip the edges of the stretcher with apprehension.

Aware that this operation is going to make me gag, I prepare the nurse, who smiles, all knowing. I take a deep breath as I watch her roll the end of the tube in lubricant. It's going to take a lot more than lubricant to push this tube up my nose and down into my stomach. Am I ready? What can I say? She places the tube into my nasal passage, obstructing my breathing, and pushes it up to the back of my nose where it meets with painful resistance. Using more force, she tries to manipulate it past the obstruction, but it doesn't move. Twisting the tube, she applies more force, which only makes my eyes tear and the inside of my nose burn. Holding the cup of water in my right hand to help me swallow the tube, I grab for some tissues with my left.

We have to take a break, while she assesses her chances of success using the other nasal passage. With more force than ease of insertion, she pushes the tube up into my nose and past the ridge. I gag uncontrollably when I drink the water that is supposed to ease the passage down to my stomach. Suddenly, I throw up all over my sweater. The nurse asks if I want to stop, but I shake my head. Since we've gone this far, I refuse to even contemplate starting over again another day. The farther she pushes the tube down, the more I seem to gag. It's getting harder to swallow the water, and each breath takes a great deal of concentration. Tears stream down my face. Finally, the nurse calmly tapes the tube into place, warning me that we have only competed the preliminaries. The tube will be advanced slowly during the x-ray.

# The Toxic Labyrinth

The radiologist, who has a great bedside manner and a marvelous sense of humor, is a bright spot in my otherwise horrific day. He slowly pushes the tube farther into my stomach, knowing that he'll stimulate the gag reflex with every move. I can see the tube in my stomach through the x-ray camera. Is it possible to move the tube through my stomach and into my small intestine? Yes it is.

My throat is so sore I can hardly swallow, but I don't want to stir. The slightest movement makes me gag. Even talking is too difficult. The enormous bag of barium hangs above me. I don't want to think about where it's going. At least I don't have to drink it. Recalling the bad memories of barium tests past, I watch the liquid drip into my gut.

The room is starting to spin. I feel restless. Nausea!! I throw up. I try to hold back. Don't throw up again. Don't throw up the tube. The barium presses against my bowel. Everyone in the room senses my distress and they encourage me to keep going. I'm ice cold and shaking. I can't feel my feet.

"Please be over," I pray. I need to move. Now my stomach is cramping, my throat aches, and I gag each time I swallow.

Thirty minutes of torture before it's finally over. Will I pass out? I'm not sure. My throat still aches even though the tube is gone. They help me off the table, but I've no strength left to stand. I need a wheelchair to get to the bathroom.

I sit on the toilet and clutch the rail for support to keep the room from spinning out of control. My legs are numb to the knees. My body can't get rid of the barium fast enough and eliminates it violently from both ends simultaneously. Where will I find the strength to leave the confines of the bathroom? God, I need to lie down.

Too weak and shaky to stand, feet and hands numb with cold, I lean on the nurse while she helps me into bed. My suspicions that the tests are making me sick have been confirmed by the morning's events.

Don peeks his head through the curtains. I try to talk. My throat is too sore to even swallow. Sympathy is visible in Don's eyes. Will a bath make me feel better? He places me in the wheelchair and organizes the soap and towels. Lovingly, he lifts me into the tub and kneeling beside it, wraps his arms around me in an effort to dispel the pain. I try to raise my arms to lather the shampoo into my hair. The motion is in vain. Gently, Don places my arms at my sides and washes my hair.

**February 24**

Although weaker than I have been all week, I have awakened feeling slightly better than yesterday. Maintaining the allergy elimination diet has allowed me to eat for the past week. This regimen should be followed for ten days, then I can increase my range of food.

Doctor G3 has just given me some amazing news. I don't now, nor did I ever have Crohn's disease. He did observe a slightly eroded area in my bowel, but it's not caused by Crohn's. I look at him in disbelief, a happy disbelief.

After I was diagnosed with this disease, I didn't exhibit most of the typical symptoms. I always wondered why I never experienced diarrhea or other symptoms common to Crohn's sufferers. Also, there was never any sign of the disease in my blood work. Chronic stomach pain was the only reason I assumed my problem was related to this disease. Have I had an allergy all these years? My stomach has always bothered me, more some days than others, depending on what I eat. If I can remedy my problem by avoiding some foods, the solution is easy.

Seven years ago, the doctor told me there was no cure, that I would be on medication for the rest of my life. I proved him wrong about the medication, which I stopped taking after four months. The medication made no difference, was costly, and violated my belief that, whenever possible, no medication is the best policy. At least I made a wise choice.

Don and I hug each other in celebration. All along I had known that the answer to my problem would be much clearer if the doctor methodically investigated my small intestine. I'm very grateful that Doctor G3 has been so thorough and given us an answer.

Before I leave, one last visit to the hospital chapel, my place of refuge far from tests and the bleakness of my room. Each day, Don has taken me to this oasis of calm. Within the confines of these walls, I have contemplated the road that lies ahead of me. Today beside the altar, I reflect on the beginnings of my spiritual awakening as an adult, a dimension of my life that has grown through my work with chronically ill children and their families.

As a caregiver, I have often formed a bond with the family during their time of crisis. When I worked in San Antonio, this attachment to the family was particularly meaningful. My children, all terminally ill, were members of families with strong internal ties. In the Hispanic culture, the family is extremely supportive and plays an integral role in the child's life. The caregiver becomes part of the extended family, a person to whom the parents look for guidance.

Although most of the families were poor, many without running water in their homes, they found ways to show their appreciation by giving me special gifts of food or homemade crafts. After the child died, often the family would return to visit with me because I was the last connection with their child. Being a part of this culture sowed the first seeds of my spiritual awakening. In my time of crisis, this gift has far greater significance than any other they could have given me.

**February 25**

As I pack, I'm ecstatic about going home. When I reflect on how sick I have been, I know I couldn't repeat my first few days here at the hospital. Although, I have been through a great deal, my final reward is wonderful. I don't have Crohn's! I'm finished with hospitals; I'm never coming back.

**February 26**

I've awakened from my sleep with nausea and dizziness. My left hand is numb. I don't want to think about symptoms. I'm home and I'm not going back to the hospital.

The flu-like feeling courses through my body and saps my strength. Mom sits with me, telling me not to be discouraged. She reminds me that after each test I felt sick until the barium was completely eliminated. A comforting thought, although physically it doesn't make me feel any better. We debate whether I should take less than a child's dosage of a laxative to eliminate the barium. Impatience wins over my no medication policy.

The laxative has started to work. My stomach is cramping, and I'm retching so hard it feels as if my insides are coming out through my mouth. The results are mixed with huge clots of blood larger than I have seen before. I lie on the bathroom floor and wonder why the sickness seems to intensify when I leave the hospital.

Mom tries to comfort me. It's been two hours since this episode started. Should I take one of the anti-nausea pills left over from my last hospital stay? My condition leaves me no choice.

We have decided to return to emergency and seek an explanation. The lights of the city shine through the car window. I would give anything to be well and out enjoying Saturday night. I've been sick far too long. Why am I not getting better? My thoughts are interrupted by Don stroking my head; he knows I need to be comforted.

The pill has calmed my severe nausea and eliminated the flu-like feeling, but my vital signs reveal low blood pressure and a low grade fever. The emergency room is busy. By the time Doctor ER4 arrives I've started to feel better. If I can drink two glasses of water, he'll send me home. A short time later, I'm on my way.

**February 28**

Only one glass of water this morning and already the gagging and retching are part of my day, and more blood clots have appeared from my bowel. Each day I'm becoming more convinced that the ranitidine, a medication that is supposed to alleviate my symptoms is making me worse.

My symptoms have been escalating all day. It's too hard to determine from my records which foods are making me sick. I'll limit myself to two or three so I can tell which ones are causing problems.

They are observing me in emergency again. My blood pressure is 76/40, but no one seems concerned.

The five hours in emergency has turned me around. My recovery periods don't form any pattern. Why are some are much shorter than others?

# CHAPTER 7

# CHANGE OF DIRECTION

An almost imperceptible light glows in the distance. I turn my exhausted, emaciated body and walk toward its faint rays.

# The Toxic Labyrinth

## March 1

Sadly, I look at the calendar. The inevitable is sinking in. It'll be some time before I'm able to work or lead a normal life. Facing the reality of not returning to Memphis, I send the notice to the apartment complex manager.

## March 2

Not only do symptoms still wake me during the night, the list increases daily. If I don't have Crohn's, and all the test results are negative, why have the symptoms not changed since my first emergency room visit last September? I dress for my follow-up appointment with Doctor G3, eat an orange, and take my medicine.

After the short drive, I felt so ill that navigating the short flight of stairs to the office was a monumental task. Now, I cower in my chair while Doctor G3 lectures me. There is no apparent reason for my multiple symptoms. He has patients with bowel cancer who don't act as sick as I do. I explain to him my stomach is burning, I'm having pain, and my bowel is eliminating clots of blood. He replies that the probable cause of the blood is piles, because my bloodwork did not reveal any abnormalities. I can barely hold up my head to look at him while he scolds me as though I were a child, and belittles me in front of Mom and Don.

After examining me, he decides to conduct a test on my stomach to check for any evidence of redness. Perhaps the symptoms at night are caused by acid reflux, and I require something stronger than ranitidine.

I argue. "I don't want the test. I had this same test in January." Mom and Don insist. I don't have any fight left. Once again I lose control.

"I can't face another test," I yell as Don half drags, half carries me to the car. Mom is angry. Why is she angry at me? I know she and Don want to believe the doctor. He sounds so reasonable. But I'm sick. Why won't anyone believe me?

"I'm not going to have the test," I tell them, my demand falling on deaf ears. I'm mad. I don't know what else to do, so I sit on the sidewalk and pound my fists, screaming that I'm going to run away. How can I run away? Trapped in a body that experiences new torments each day, I'm too sick to look after myself. I just want to give up.

Mom pulls me from the sidewalk. "Get into the car." I sit facing the window and cry all the way home.

"I'm not going into the apartment. I'm staying in the car."

I sit in the car, the only place I can be alone, and cry. There's no privacy with four people living in a one bedroom apartment. I have no space, no place that is mine. It is worthless to even speculate about running away when I don't have any money or the energy to walk up a short flight of stairs.

Mom has come back to talk with me. "Heather, I know it's hard for you. I'm sorry I was angry, but I can't let you quit. We have to make sure there is nothing in your stomach. This is the doctor that proved you never had Crohn's. Let's see what he finds tomorrow."

I'm defiant. If there's nothing wrong with me, then it doesn't matter what I do. I eat some more oranges to prove my point. Eventually, I surrender and return to the apartment, angry and unrepentant.

As the night closes in, my body succumbs to the next barrage. The demons are back, accompanied by an unquenchable thirst. I lie on the bed wondering why my body doesn't give up and die. Death seems the only reasonable escape at times like this. No one understands how hellish it is to be in my body. The sickness is making me restless. I writhe, tears from the pain streaming down my face. Don holds my hand while I try to express my thoughts.

# The Toxic Labyrinth

"I can't take this any more," I tell him. "I want the angels to come and take me. I can't endure living inside this body day after day."

Don offers soft words of encouragement. "You can't give up. If we keep searching for the answer, eventually we'll be successful. You have to keep fighting." Watching his face as he strokes my hair and wipes away my tears, I can tell he feels as helpless as I do.

Sometime during the long night, my body deals with the demons, and sleep comes to the rescue.

## March 3

Morning has brought the quiet illusion of relief. Eating is not permitted before the test, and so I take a leisurely bath. While drying my face, I look in the mirror at my neck. The crimson, itching rash triggers memories of the one I had in Memphis. Didn't I take the ranitidine just fifteen minutes ago? Severe gagging and nausea interrupt my thoughts, confirming my theory that the medicine is aggravating my symptoms.

Later, as I slowly change into the hospital gown, I shudder. I hate all of this, the hospital and the testing. It's so degrading. I've become no more than a thorn in the side of medicine, a faceless entity with no choice and no voice, constantly at the mercy of people who don't believe me.

The long, thick, black scope will soon be down my throat. I shudder. The mouth guard slips between my teeth. My eyes follow the syringe to the injection site. I'm still conscious when the tech directs me to swallow. Someone far away is gagging. Mercifully blackness triumphs.

The low reading on the blood pressure machine slides into focus. Is the nurse monitoring me? Blackness again.

Doctor G3 has returned with the results. Although my stomach is red, the ranitidine will heal whatever is causing the irritation. I thank him politely for taking time with me and leave as quickly as possible. Free from the tentacles of the testing room, I vow never to return.

To add some enjoyment to our rather bleak existence, Don and I attend a play at a nearby theater. The seat at the back, high up and away from the crowd makes me less claustrophobic. How exciting to be out on a date. As the plot unfolds, I become agitated and restless. My chest tightens, and I repeatedly shift my position, rocking back and forth for comfort, determined to stay until the end.

Although tired during the walk back home, I'm much improved after leaving the theater.

**March 4**

Mom has returned from her walk armed with a number of books on food allergy, and has laid them out on the bed. As I start to read, I realize that my knowledge is limited. How does one define food intolerance, a new concept to me? Apparently, there are no reliable tests to indicate if food allergies or intolerance are present. Is this a key to my negative test results? I read on. The immune system is involved; the reason is not really understood. There are varying degrees of and terms for adverse food reactions. Reactions can build. One can eat a small amount of a food and have a minimum reaction, but if the food is eaten later the same day, the reaction can be much more pronounced. Eating the same food three days in a row may cause a reaction only on the fourth day.

I remember the oranges I ate two days ago. Referring to my records, I confirm my suspicions about their effect. Obviously, my reactions at the doctor's office and later in the day were directly related to the oranges. Looking over the list of adverse food reactions, I realize it includes all the symptoms I've been experiencing: numbness, confusion, hives, stomach problems, nausea, asthma, and many more. There is a withdrawal phenomenon that occurs when an allergy causing food is taken out of the diet. After the food is eliminated, it can take from five to twenty days to clear the effects. This theory makes sense. My improvement after a week on IV is relative to the time it takes to clear my symptoms. Like an addict, I experience withdrawal symptoms, sensations associated with the elimination of the offending foods. The cycle of withdrawal starts on the first day and reaches a peak on the third or fourth day. One of my withdrawal symptoms is the burning back pain that occurs during the first days on IV treatment and subsides after a few days. Maybe I'm getting closer to the answer.

Reading about elimination diets and the benefit of discovering problematic foods helps me establish a course of action. It's time to take control. First, I'll stop the ranitidine because medication interferes with proper evaluation of allergies. Besides, I suspect this medication has been adding to my problems.

I've stopped the ranitidine and started drinking distilled water, causing the low back pain to recur. Nevertheless, I've prepared myself to feel worse for the first few days and will just have to work through the symptoms.

**March 6**

The last few days were filled with horrendous symptoms, too numerous to record accurately. I concentrated only on those which caused major discomfort.

Drinking clear fluids brought about oppressive hunger and extreme nausea, one alternating with the other. The multitude of symptoms, combined with constant agitation, made it impossible to concentrate on the TV, divert my mind with games, or read.

During my first night without the ranitidine, the agitation and aching in my back kept me from sleeping. Incessant thirst caused me to drink continually, my hands and feet alternated between ice cold and red hot, my ears rang, and the flu-like symptoms continued unabated.

By the third day the symptoms were continuous and seemed endless. What started out as a normal morning soon escalated into a nightmare with symptoms coming in waves, each wave followed by a short clear period. My face alternated between its normal pallor and beet red. Obviously, the ranitidine had masked even more than my usual complement of symptoms.

That night, I spent hours praying for relief when the nausea and waves of symptoms became almost intolerable. Mom and Don tried to persuade me to take a very small amount of anti-nausea medication, but I resisted. I knew the drug could be habit forming.

Don lay beside me, rubbing my back for hours, trying to calm the agitation in a body too sick to respond to his touch. Finally, I surrendered and took the pill. The rage inside my body had won. Relief, the first I'd had in three days, lulled me to sleep.

**March 7**

It's time to renew the relationship with my regular family physician, Doctor John, whom I haven't seen for eighteen months. When I first arrived in Vancouver, Grace managed my care. Because we had been in contact while I was ill in Memphis, and she knew my history, calling her first was a natural decision. Once I was in the health care system and involved with the specialists, my family doctor didn't fit into the pattern of care. Now that my condition has become chronic, Grace and I have decided that my family physician should oversee my care. I had wanted to make contact with him when I wasn't in a crisis state, and had hoped to appear somewhat lively for our initial meeting.

I lean against Don's shoulder in the doctor's office, expecting to find some comfort. The office staff are concerned by my appearance and immediately prepare an examining room. Relieved that I don't have to hold up my head, I lie on the examining table and relate my medical history. Without interrupting, Doctor John listens to the synopsis of events over the past five months and our present conclusions. His concern is evident. Rarely have I required medical advice, even for my Crohn's. My usual visit to him in the past was precipitated by a new 'traveler' assignment. We would laugh and crack jokes while he wrote the note verifying I was healthy enough to work outside Canada. Today there are no jokes.

While Doctor John consults his medical books, he mentions a friend who has been very ill because of allergies. The shot I received in Memphis to enhance my immune system elicits many questions. What kind of reaction did I have after the injection? He looks up serum sickness. A possibility. I have all the signs.

My thoughts drift back to the children I cared for on the cancer unit. To boost their immune systems, they were injected with substances which caused reactions similar to mine. Each day I'm being pulled further into their world.

Doctor John's instructions to Don capture my attention. "Take Heather to the emergency room for fluids. I will phone ahead so they will expect you. The IV fluids will perk her up, until she feels well enough to eat again."

He's listening to me!

The wait at emergency has been over an hour. Don's coat forms a makeshift bed on the floor. My body presses against the cold, concrete floor of the waiting room as I move my hip to find some comfort in this inhospitable environment. My mind floats in and out, the frantic sounds of people and ambulances blurring into an incomprehensible discord.

I don't want to relate my story to Doctor ER5. My stomach is cramping, and I have a desperate urge to drink. I just want the IV. How reliant I have become on this procedure over the last few months.

The nurse slips the catheter in with ease and opens the clamp wide. Can my abused body tolerate the fluid at such a fast rate? But there's no need to worry, it sucks up the fluid like a sponge. The agitation slips away and the cramping in my stomach fades.

To pass the time, Don and I play hang man. We are in the middle of a game when a sudden cold invades my body, causing me to shake violently. Closing the roller clamp on the IV tubing a little, I call the nurse who, noticing my distress, takes my vital signs. "Your blood pressure is a little low. You really need these IV fluids."

Don holds my hand until the shaking subsides. By the time the second bag of fluid is half finished, I am relaxed enough to drift off to sleep. The rest and the fluids give me the energy to leave the emergency room with little assistance from Don.

I crawl into bed, thanking God I have found a doctor who seems to believe me. Buoyed up by the fluids and my good luck, I fall asleep in good spirits.

**March 9**

Doctor John has arranged for me to see an allergist, Doctor A2. I had called a Seattle allergy clinic in January, but the first available appointment wasn't until in June. Now, I don't have to wait. This direction seems to hold the answer. I have high hopes.

Mom and I sit in Doctor A2's office surrounded by my ever expanding medical documents, which are now contained in a file and a binder. He takes an unusual and sketchy history, telling me repeatedly to keep the information brief because he is not interested in details. The fact he opposes food testing is seconded by me. No more injections until my body stabilizes.

I convey my concerns about lack of nutrition and request the name of a dietitian who specializes in allergies. He brushes aside my request by remarking that I don't require dietary assistance, yet. He instructs me to make another appointment after he has conferred with Doctor G3, and dismisses me.

Mom and I leave the office in a state of confusion and apprehension. I'm depending on this man to help me. Does he really understand the seriousness of my condition?

## March 11

Time alone with Don is precious. To spend a few days by ourselves, we have planned a weekend in the heart of the city, close to Mom's apartment and the hospitals. We are being cautious this time.

A view of the mountains and harbor compensates for the cubicle which passes for a luxury suite. The cooler in the corner of our room is packed with my special food. Down the hall, paint cans and building materials are stacked, waiting for workers to finish renovations. Even though the situation isn't idyllic, nothing can spoil our romantic weekend.

Hand in hand, we explore the pleasures of Robson: stores filled with the latest spring fashions, gourmet restaurants beckoning our senses with different ethnic foods. We've descended to the bottom of the street which is several blocks long. Symptoms are nagging in the background. I look up toward the hotel. Do my legs have the strength to make the climb? I lean on Don and cry with frustration as he assists me up the hill and back to the room.

"It's just not fair. I don't understand why I can't predict these sick spells. I'm a prisoner. I want out of this body."

Don offers patient words of consolation. "If you rest tonight maybe you'll be better tomorrow."

"The shops are located up the hill from the hotel? We have made special arrangements for our last weekend together, and I can't walk up the hill. How am I going to shop and see the sights?"

"We've made progress this weekend just leaving the apartment. If you don't feel well, I'll drive you the few blocks up the hill." Don puts his arms around me, wipes away my tears, and seals his promise with a hug.

**March 12**

Just a few symptoms, which I can live with this morning. After my breakfast of lamb and yams, we are on our way. The sun is bathing the city with its warmth, and I celebrate its energy. Determined to climb the two blocks to the shops, I don't need the car. On the crest of the hill, I stand looking at the hotel far below me. "Heather, the conqueror," I congratulate myself silently.

Don has no interest men's fashion, a personal expenditure he finds wasteful and foolish. We tease him constantly about his wardrobe, a mishmash of items thrown together for their utility, not their style. One pair of patterned lounging pants, which we refer to as his 'clown pants', are so garish that his employer declared them unsuitable for meetings, even in remote areas of Nigeria. However, when it comes to my wardrobe, he is indulgent and generous. Today he comments that my thirty-pound weight loss makes my clothes hang. It looks like I'm wearing his pants, and so it's time for new jeans. Normally, I would be ecstatic with the new slim me. Under the circumstances, I am nervous about the rapid weight loss. Most of the time, I'm too preoccupied with my health to enjoy my new figure.

I'm in a fog. Why is my mind reacting this way? I leave the dressing room quickly to purchase the jeans and leave the store. Out on the street, the feeling passes, and I'm ready for more adventures.

Back in the hotel, I rejoice at my accomplishments. I've completed a two-hour shopping and walking trip. A perfect day, except that my eyes burn when I'm in the hotel room.

# The Toxic Labyrinth

## March 13

A glorious day spent lounging on the grass in the park and walking around the seawall. With each minute I seem to improve. Even my temperature is normal. The only gray edge to this marvelous day is Don's imminent departure.

I'm brave enough to talk about the future now that I'm improving. Our marriage, which I have refused to consider during the last few months, is a possibility once more. October is a reasonable choice, because Don will be home and I'll have enough time to plan. We cuddle on a log facing the ocean and dream about the wedding. It's a wonderful day to be in love.

## March 14

Usually Don and I are alone in the car when I drive him to the airport. Today Mom has to drive us because I don't feel confident enough to manage on my own. Despondent, I say good-bye for another month. Not wanting to display my emotions, I hold back my tears on the return trip. It isn't easy, even at the best of times, being the one left behind.

I have added broccoli and potatoes to my food list, trying to eat them at least four hours apart so I can determine if either of them causes a reaction.

Gossiping and sharing a few laughs, Melodie and I visit in a small cafe after our shopping trip. Gradually, my interest in our afternoon dissipates. The flu-like feeling, absent for the last few days, is creeping back.

It's almost 5 p.m. My left arm is hurting, sections of my face are tingling and numb, the roof of my mouth feels swollen, and the back of my neck is burning. I cry as I look back at my records to determine the offending food. My notes seem to indicate potatoes as the culprit. I decide to revert to the diet of lamb, yams, and rice which gave me such energy on the weekend.

Mom sits beside me uttering words of encouragement. "Heather, you are doing very well. Don't get discouraged. You know, life is full of surprises. Maybe the days ahead will bring more good things."

"Do you have any plans for Wednesday?" she asks.

"Plans? I don't make plans these days."

"I'm expecting a package and may not be home. Can you be here to answer the door?"

"Yes, I'll be here," I reply.

My sadness is building each day, and I need to vent my private, depressing thoughts. How can anyone who has not had the experience understand the agony of being ill for months? I pick up the tape recorder Don has given me and articulate my thoughts.

"What do I want the most? I want to be well. I want to stop being afraid of everything. I'm afraid to go anywhere by myself. I'm afraid I'll be too sick to help myself. I never know when the bouts of sickness will strike. There is no rhyme nor reason to much of what has happened to me.

"Today I was afraid to drive Don to the airport. Who is this person? This isn't me. I want to be able to do all the things I used to do. I want to be able to go for long walks by myself and not get tired or be afraid of needing help. I want a day with no symptoms. No wrist pain. No joint pain. No tingling or numbness. I want to feel normal. I want to have my old energy back.

"I want to visit my grandmothers. I want to have a normal relationship with Don, one that does not always focus on my illness.

"I want to go to the bathroom normally without watching blood and mucous pour out of my bowel. I want to eat in a restaurant. I want to drink milk. I want to go for a swim. I want to be able to work. There are so many things I took for granted that I want to be able to do again. Patience and prayer are now my constant companions.

# The Toxic Labyrinth

"Maybe I will never be completely well again. I think of that often. Maybe there is no positive future for me. I am so sad and afraid. I cry every day. Sometimes I feel so alone because no one can really know how I feel inside."

I put down the recorder and turn off the light.

## March 16

Eating foods low on the allergy scale is not helping. My symptoms still persist. I'm trying to keep accurate records, but it's difficult to determine what foods are making me so sick. After eleven days on the elimination diet, I had hoped for an improvement; I must need more time.

While I can sit up, I'm downstairs in Mom's office working on medical bills, a task I can't leave until the next day. I never know what tomorrow will bring.

The doorbell sounds and expecting delivery of Mom's parcel, I open the door.

"Hi, Heath."

I'm speechless. Rhonda, my sister, is standing in the hallway. She's supposed to be in England. My mind is working in slow motion, trying to assimilate the moment. I stand in disbelief, leaving Rhonda to struggle with her suitcase. Suddenly, I realize she is not an illusion and embrace her, my tears of happiness spilling onto her jacket. Mom had planned this surprise for me. The parcel she was expecting is my sister, whom I haven't seen in a year.

Rhonda and I lie in the dark talking quietly while I pour out my frustration and fears. Rhonda calmly assesses the situation.

"I know you are going to get well, Heather. That's why I haven't been home until now. Getting better will be the hardest thing you will ever have to do. I think there is some purpose for your illness, a purpose you will comprehend in the future."

Rhonda's words are soothing yet disturbing.

# Change of Direction

"Have you considered alternative forms of medicine? I've told you before, there are lots of other ways to go besides conventional medicine."

Rhonda and I have been communicating weekly since my first hospitalization. In her letters and telephone calls she has been urging me to seek out methods of assistance other than conventional western medicine. Rhonda speaks from experience. She has used different forms of therapy to lessen her chronic neck pain. Her words have given me something to think about.

**March 17**

Because my symptoms are escalating, I have made another appointment with Doctor John. He encourages me to keep going and maintain my regimen. Despite the return of my symptoms, and my ability to eat only a few foods, he thinks I'm going in the right direction and promises to keep track of my declining weight.

Rhonda and I are going to a movie with Jane. I don't want them to know I had trouble walking to the car, so I rest silently in the back seat, conserving my strength while Jane and Rhonda catch up with their news. Even conversing is too strenuous for me, and I'm grateful that Jane has Rhonda to talk to.

I try to match my stride when we walk toward the theater, but with each step, I meet resistance. As the images move across the screen, claustrophobia winds its wily arms around me, arms that slowly close around my chest, squeezing. Agitated and unable to focus on the movie, I move in my seat. It's no use. I have to leave.

Once again, I have to rely on someone to take care of me. Bob has brought me home from the movie and will stay with me until Mom arrives home. Tonight, I don't want to be left alone.

# The Toxic Labyrinth

## March 22

The day has started badly. I lie in bed, cringing as the symptoms wash over me. A new symptom has added its pattern to my torment. I now have difficulty moving my jaw.

Why is no one is home? I'm afraid to get out of bed. When I move around, the symptoms intensify. I switch on the recorder:

"Nothing has changed. Not only am I reacting to the food I eat, my reactions seem to be continuous. There is no way to time them. My tongue feels numb and paralyzed. Will I choke while I'm chewing? I can't grip anything with my left hand. Am I having little strokes? My legs hurt so much I can't touch my legs when I bathe. I'm afraid. I only weigh one hundred and twenty-six pounds. I began this battle at one hundred and sixty-two pounds. There is not much more weight to lose. I pray everyday.

"I attempt to make plans, which I can rarely keep or follow through to the end. I will not make plans anymore. Don and I had planned to travel to Hawaii and Louisiana during his next month home, but I can't go. I'm losing hope. Every day runs into the next, bringing more disappointments and even more symptoms.

"I've been sick for one hundred and seventy-three days. The year will end, and nothing will change. I wake up in the morning feeling slightly better, and by the end of the day I'm sick again. I cry every day. Please help me God."

I lash out at Rhonda and Mom. "Where have you been? Why did you leave me alone?"

"We went for a walk so Rhonda could spend a little time with me before she leaves tomorrow. We weren't gone that long," Mom says.

But I refuse to be pacified, even though I know my attitude is selfish and unreasonable. The fear of what might happen to me, when I least expect it, is too powerful to be conquered by common sense.

I'm so discouraged. The new foods, sweet potatoes, spinach and turkey, are no better than the rest.

The end of the day has brought some relief. The unbearable ache in my ribs and my legs has disappeared.

## March 23

The walk from the airport parking lot has sapped my energy. How can I visit with Rhonda until she disappears through security? As we search around for a solution, my glance falls on the cart carrying Rhonda's baggage. I perch on the bottom rack of the luggage cart while Mom pushes me around the airport. The other passengers look at the rather weird trio, but we are not fazed. More and more we are learning to be creatures of our own destiny, rather than follow the dictates of society.

On our way back from the airport, we have stopped at a store which sells food for allergy sufferers. Mom and I read the labels to decide what food would expand my range of carbohydrates. Since rice now causes a reaction, my intake of carbohydrates is very limited, and taking in enough calories each day is becoming more difficult.

## March 24

I slept through the night, and that fact starts the day on a positive note.

Another food that isn't working. I was feeling relatively well until I ate my last piece of venison. Now the agitation and the flu-like symptoms have returned. Even the burning in the back of my neck has progressed to headaches and a tingling that pulses up and down my back.

Mom has cooked the tapioca—a muck resembling fish eggs—that we bought yesterday as a substitute for rice. At best it looks unappetizing, but this is not the issue. I have to be able to eat the stuff. Three tablespoons down the hatch. The room is becoming foggy. My esophagus is burning and my face is numb, right into my mouth. The violent pain shooting into my left arm takes me by surprise. I sit on the sofa shaking, my teeth chattering.

"Mom," I call.

"What's wrong?"

"The tapioca is making me feel really strange. Like I'm going to pass out."

Mom holds me until the shaking stops. Tapioca is not something I will be trying again soon. What am I going to do? I'm not getting enough to eat. Because I was overweight when my illness began, no one, except me, seems concerned about my lack of calories. My situation is getting worse instead of better. Most of what I eat produces a reaction and symptoms. My situations seem impossible. Each day, I'm getting thinner and weaker from lack of nutrition. Even though I'm expanding my knowledge about allergies, I think I'm beyond any help these books can give me.

Reviewing my food charts shows a nutritional decline to an average of eight hundred calories a day. My body is starving. I have to find a source of carbohydrate I can eat without getting sick. My situation is getting desperate.

**March 25**

Every day is a struggle. Lack of carbohydrates is only one of my problems. I think I have other nutritional deficiencies as well. I really need some form of supplement. I need help and I need it now.

My attempts at finding assistance seem to be foiled at each turn. My plan to visit an allergist in Seattle was canceled because I'm too weak to travel. My appointment at a local clinic, which I made in February, is not until the end of April. Desperate for even minimal information, I dial the local clinic and speak with the receptionist.

Explaining my crisis state, I beg her to help me. What does the clinic recommend for patients who can't eat anything? After much persuasion, she mentions that even their sickest patients can tolerate Formula.

This is a product I trust. My children who could not tolerate any food were fed Formula, a liquid that has all the nutrients in proportion. Because the nutrients are predigested, Formula is absorbed at the beginning of the small intestine. I send Mom out to buy a trial package.

After we have mixed Formula according to the instructions for regular use, I sip the mixture, gagging on each mouthful. The smell is absolutely revolting and reminds me of caring for debilitated patients. I put a lid on the cup to minimize the odor. Diluting the solution with water makes it more palatable.

Two hours have passed. I'm shaking violently and uncontrollably. Mom and Doug have just left for a walk, and frantically, I call her on the cellular.

"Come back. I don't not know what's happening."

I call Doctor John's office. But I reach a doctor on call who is not familiar with my case. There is nothing to do except wait and hope the symptoms will subside.

The shaking has finally stopped. What's happening to my body? What's happening to my life? Why is God refusing me the answer, or is he teaching me patience by giving me the solution in small pieces?

As the day progresses, the energy that flows into my body eliminates the numbness in my hands. Although I have a headache and my thirst is back, I'm so much better. Is this a sign that Formula is giving me the nutrients I have been lacking? I dilute it even more and slowly sip throughout the evening, not understanding why my thirst increases with each drink.

# The Toxic Labyrinth

## March 26

Another restless night. I've awakened for the second time tonight and started to shake, part of the pattern of more frequent sleeplessness. I'm cold, agitated, and my bones ache. It's difficult to decide what's making me sick. The symptoms are random, forming no pattern, and even spacing out foods during the day to establish a trend, reveals little consistency. There is no trend; my symptoms are incessant.

Instead of rolling fitfully around in bed, I've decided to drink more Formula. Carefully diluting the mixture by four times the instructions, I sip it while eating a small helping of yams. The yams soon make me gag and retch. As the nausea hits full force, my hands and stomach cramp and the thirst is unbearable. I brace myself against a weakness that is pushing me toward unconsciousness.

At 7 a.m. I wake Mom. "You have to take me to the emergency room. I need some fluids."

Gagging nonstop into a basin tucked between my knees and drinking continuously, I wait for a bed in emergency. Everything is spinning; I need that IV.

The nurse takes my vital signs. Knowing the details of the last six months will be too confusing, I relate a short history, just enough to get the IV. A few months ago, I dreaded this procedure. Now I welcome the stab as it brings the relief of soothing fluids. While the IV works its miracle, I drink as fast as I can to quench my thirst.

Doctor ER6 listens to my story. Unlike the typical emergency room physician I've encountered, he listens intently. He agrees to check my blood to determine whether everything is in balance. My flank pain and unexplained fever concern him, and he also wants to check my urine for infection. The thought of this test, which requires a catheter directly into the bladder to collect an uncontaminated sample, makes me cringe.

The nurse is very caring and skilled, but the procedure is still uncomfortable and humbling. I lie on the table, legs spread wide apart while the urine drains through the catheter. Even though I'm unable to quench my thirst, my body is beginning to eliminate the IV fluids.

Have I ever been a nurse? I've been the patient for such a long time.

Although the first set of tests are normal, my excessive thirst is unusual, and the doctor suggests checking for diabetes and thyroid malfunction. Leafing through a medical book, he quizzes me further about my symptoms. We discuss the possibility of another gastroenterologist to solve my problem, and he recommends one who always deals with the intractable cases. Although he is certain this doctor will find answers, I share my apprehension with him about taking this route.

Delving further into my problem, he discusses my fears about eating and, at the same time, encourages me to eat. Have I considered the possibility of anorexia? The word strikes a chord deep within me; I don't have that, do I? My symptoms are real. He talks further about the importance of conquering my fear of food, although he's not certain this is my problem. As he prepares to leave, he gives me some last advice.

"Heather, keep an open mind and don't get desperate," he says kindly. This doctor has spent most of the morning with me, discussing my case and being supportive, and this is something I have not experienced with any other emergency room physician. He's a wonderful man. I'll have to think about his words.

Mom and I have decided to see what happens if I eat normally. I have started with steak, bananas, asparagus, sweet potatoes, and cantaloupe. I'm going to eat anything I want. But the symptoms not only continue, they have escalated. My legs ache with cold up into my knees. I'm weak and my left arm is numb. I continue to eat and nothing changes. By the end of the evening the burning in the back of my neck is intense, and I ache everywhere. Waves of symptoms wash over me continually.

# The Toxic Labyrinth

"Mom, why is it taking so long to find the answer? Today, I've been sick for one hundred and eighty days."

"Heather, one hundred and eighty degrees is half way around a circle. Maybe these next few days will be a turning point for you." Mom is always so optimistic.

## March 27

Despite my symptoms, I've slept through the night. Encouraged by Mom and the bright day, I have decided to go for a ride. We sit in the car watching the sea gulls dip and dive for food in the shallow water.

"Heather, you can't give up. There's a future out there for you. We just can't see it yet." Mom is trying to convince me that it's important to go on, to keep trying.

"We both have to get on with our lives before this problem consumes us. Somehow you have to conquer your fear of being alone and your dependence on me. You keep to yourself, more and more. Each time your friends and even when your grandmothers call, you want me to take a message, so you don't have to talk to them."

But my life has degenerated into trips to the hospital and a concern for my health. I used to have an exciting life, one that my friends envied. Now I'm an object of pity. This conversation only reinforces my fear of what is to come and the imposition I have been on Mom's life for many months. I cry. I yell. I feel like I'm going crazy.

As we start screaming at each other, I try to get out of the car. "I'm going to walk home."

"You can't walk home, Heather. You can barely ride in the car." Mom grabs me by the hair to keep me from leaving.

"No one understands how sick I am. I feel like hell inside," I yell.

# Change of Direction

We cry and yell, our voices resounding though the car and into the parking lot. I knew the time would come when Mom would need a break. I want a break, too. Where do I go?

She's right. I'm pushing all the people close to me away. I don't want to phone my friends any more. What do I have to talk about, nothing except being sick and going to the doctor.

"You have so much to look forward to. This will pass. Although it seems you have been sick for a long time, in the whole span of your life, it's a short time. I won't stand by and watch you give up."

I don't want to listen to Mom's words; I just want to die.

Our yelling has subsided. "Mom, you need a break. I'll stay with Dad for a while."

"That won't work. Your Dad is too far from your doctor and the hospital. Heather, look at the sunshine today. The winter was so dull. It rained almost every day. The sun is finally starting to shine. Maybe all the very sick children you cared for are smiling down, telling you that things will change."

Mom's words strike a chord. In our material world, we become less spiritual until we are faced with a crisis that seems beyond solution by mere mortals and we turn to a higher level of comfort. Are my children trying to take care of me like I took care of them? Do those who have gone before have the power to help us? Is Grandpa, who was a doctor, looking down from Heaven and communicating with us in subtle ways? Sometimes I think he is conveying the answers, but we are unable to see the whole picture.

Our anger and frustration spent for the moment, Mom and I hug each other and determine to enjoy the rest of our drive. During the ride home, we hide our true feelings behind cheerful conversation.

My former roommate, Brian, has dropped in unexpectedly on his way through the city. He is an old friend, so I am making an effort at conversation. We roomed together when he was studying medicine. At the time, I was working as a nurse and would scoff at any suggestion he might know more than I did. How could he, a lowly student, be as informed as someone who had hospital experience? Now times have changed, and I pour out my tale of woe to Dr. Brian.

"Heather, just because they can't find anything wrong with you, doesn't mean you're not sick. Maybe the test hasn't been invented yet, to diagnose what you are experiencing or maybe they aren't looking for the right cause."

For the moment, listening to Brian has raised my level of confidence. As a doctor and a friend, he has validated my condition. Little does he realize how important his opinion and reassurance is in strengthening my resolve to beat this thing.

Later, while Mom tries to comfort me during one of my episodes, she looks through a nutrition book for answers.

"Heather, your Grandpa gave me this book a number of years ago. He believed in building up the body, in making it strong enough to withstand illness. One of the reasons I fed you balanced meals and didn't give you sugar as a child was the result of what he taught me."

"Mom, I was thinking about Grandpa today. Because we keep returning to look at this book for answers, I want you to tell me some more about him."

"Grandpa was an old fashioned family doctor, who made house calls. He often knew several generations of a family, which made it much easier to diagnose their aches and pains. Do you remember his favorite saying?" Mom asks.

"Yes. 'Always listen to the patient.' Now everything is done with tests and pills."

"His words keep coming back to me whenever you tell me about your symptoms. They always seem to be related to the time of day and what you have eaten or the medicine you have taken."

I start to cry. I want to believe that Grandpa is telling us what to do through the people who are involved in our lives. Was he giving us directions through Doctor ER6, who took so much time with me yesterday? Maybe Grandpa is listening. I have to keep praying.

Today, I tried to eat different foods than I did yesterday: pork, melon, apple, and wild rice. I'm trying to rotate foods, so that I don't build up an intolerance. The plan isn't working. I'm nauseated and having difficulty moving my left hand; the glands in my neck are swelling and the constant thirst is increasing.

**March 28**

I'm plunging deeper into this sickness. My agitated body won't let me sleep for any length of time, and I lie in my bed restless, and shaking. Each time I wake, I try to eat. My thirst is unquenchable, and I'm voiding every half hour. What is happening?

It's 4 a.m., and Mom lies beside me, holding me while I retch and shake.

"Try and hang on until we can call Doctor John in the morning. There's no use going to the emergency room. They will just send you home again."

The constant thirst is making me drink too much fluid, and I try to limit my intake. I'm exhausted, but I can't sleep.

Finally it's 8:00 a.m. No night in my life has been longer. As I throw up in the bathroom, I hear Mom making arrangements for me to see Doctor John immediately.

In Doctor John's office, I retch while Mom explains my situation. He consults his medical books. Maybe I have a rare condition called diabetes insipidous. Agreeing that my condition is serious, he arranges for a hospital admission under an internist whom he thinks may be able to help.

Doctor John's office has called to say there will be no bed until tomorrow. If I think it will help, I can to the emergency for more IV fluids.

# The Toxic Labyrinth

This condition is like an addiction, requiring a fix of IV fluids every few days. My head is too heavy to hold up, and I lie across several chairs in the waiting room. Mom wants me to sit up. She is worried I will give the impression of anxiety, and the emergency staff won't deal with me. I can hear the frustration in her voice, see the fatigue in her face. Just leave me in the hospital to die. I'm not getting better. There are no answers. It's a vicious circle I can't go around any more. The emergency room staff make it quite clear I'm only allowed to have fluids. I can't be admitted. Sick as I am, I have to wait for a bed.

I look up in surprise to see that Doctor John has come to the emergency room. He says it's important for me to be admitted tomorrow. I nod in agreement, unable gather the strength for conversation.

"How do you feel?" he asks.

"Like hell," I answer. I want to be more pleasant with someone who has taken the time to see me, but I can't.

Questions and more questions. "Why are you not being admitted by Doctor G2?" Doctor ER7 asks. "Are you working?" I know exactly what he's implying and I'm getting so tired of defending myself.

"Haven't I seen you before?" he asks this question twice.

"No," I say. I honestly don't remember him until after he leaves. His is just one of dozens of faces I've seen during the last six months. I hate the emergency room. The IV can't finish soon enough, so I can return home.

Desperate, Mom believes we must discover more information about foods I can possibly eat. Using a list of dietitians, she has phoned each one seeking information. Finally, she has located one who understands the critical nature of my condition and will phone the local allergy clinic to intervene on my behalf.

Putting down the phone, Mom shares her good news. "Doctor Joan, the nutritionist and dietitian, at the clinic will see me tomorrow.

Even though, you will be in the hospital, she will discuss a method of action with me." I'm not certain what can be done, but it's worth a try.

I stare at the picture of my Grandpa in Mom's office, crying and begging him to give me the answer. This whole mess is so stressful. It's hard on me and now it's starting to affect my family. I have nowhere else to go. I hate infringing on Mom's life and her space. What else can I do? I'm not well enough to stay at my Dad's. This time I'm not leaving the hospital until there is a solution.

I phone Don to tell him I want to give up. I can't stop crying. What can he do or say when he is so far away, except listen and give me words of encouragement.

**March 29**

The shaking is unremitting. Too agitated to sleep or watch TV, I sit on my bed and rock back and forth. I gulp down water as fast as I can to quench my persisting and increasing thirst. Two nights without sleep, and tonight will be no different. Every few minutes I look at the clock, watching the hours drag.

"Please let it be morning."

Finally, at 3:30 a.m. I can't stand it anymore and call Bob who agreed earlier to take me to the hospital. Grabbing the bag I have packed, I look one last time at the picture of my Grandpa. "Please, let this be the last time I have to go to the hospital," I plead. The photograph has captured his laughing, loving eyes, the way they always were when I was a little girl. Is he in Heaven listening to my plea?

Bob has stopped at an all-night convenience store to buy me a bottle of water. I have already finished what I had brought with me. I look out the window into the blackness of the early morning. How could my life have come to this? One day I was leading a happy and fascinating life, the next I was entrenched in the health care system.

## The Toxic Labyrinth

What has happened to the woman I used to be? Now I'm a slave to my body and the hospital. Is there no escape? I bow my head to hide the tears from Bob.

I feel another hand covering my right hand. The touch brings a feeling of comfort and serenity, a premonition that everything will be all right. I look up. The feeling vanishes. I look at Bob who is concentrating on the road. He is sitting on my left, and I had felt the hand on my right side. Did I imagine the whole thing? The incident was so real. Is someone else here with us? I shake my head and attribute the whole incident to my illness.

Doctor ER8 is annoyed and asks condescending questions. What can he possibly do for me at 4 a.m.? I tell him repeatedly about my insatiable thirst. He asks me how long it's been since I have worked, making me feel even more sick and degraded. Finally, he agrees to check if there is an order to admit me. Admitting hasn't registered my bed, and it will be 8 a.m. before someone can correct the error. Doctor ER8 has refused to start an IV, but insists that I sit in emergency until my bed is ready. I've so little energy left to fight this illness, and certainly no excess to continually defend myself against those who don't believe. I'm so sick inside, yet the tests don't show physical signs. I don't understand.

I lie on my bed with the door closed, shutting out the hospital sounds and drinking in the tranquillity of my sanctuary. I realize that I haven't been alone since November. The private room will give me time to reflect on where I'm going and whether I have the strength to continue the fight.

The internist, Doctor Joe, disturbs my thoughts. During his examination, I decide to focus on my joint pains. Even though the numbness is a more distressing symptom, doctors don't equate joint pain with psychiatric problems. If I have to, I'll alter my history to avoid being locked away. Doctor Joe is a very nice man who listens. Does he believe that I have allergy problems? First he'll contact the allergist and the hospital dietitian.

## Change of Direction

Just when I think I can't stand the symptoms another minute, there is a window of calm while the waves of horrendous discomfort wash away.

The nurse enters with my IV solution. Checking the solution, I note it's not the usual type. The IV nurse is familiar. I've spent so much of the year in hospitals, I'm beginning to recognize the staff. I remember this nurse specifically. She missed twice when she started my IV the last time. Hopefully, today will not be a repeat of our last meeting.

Dad and Bob are with me. I'm following the usual pattern. I've stopped eating and the regenerating fluids are dripping into my vein, making me well enough to visit.

The nurse has returned with an IV bag which is yellow in color. I ask about the contents. Doctor Joe has given her orders to add vitamins to the IV. I'm uncertain about this decision, but the vitamins will give me the nutrition I desperately need. I continue to visit, my mind on other matters.

While Dad finds something to eat, Bob keeps me company. My thirst, which had almost subsided, has returned. Restless and agitated, I shift around on the bed, hoping Bob will carry the conversation. I'm losing my ability to think about anything else except how horrible I feel.

"Bob, I feel ill. I need more to drink. This IV is drying my eyes." The room is getting hazy and I'm starting to shake. The nausea comes out of nowhere. I have to throw up. I reach over and turn off the IV.

The attending nurse is young and inexperienced, so I have to control the situation, insisting that the solution has to be changed because I can't tolerate it. Thirst is causing me to drink so much fluid, my stomach can't hold it all. She calls in a senior nurse who decides to leave the IV turned off until she hears from the doctor.

The nausea has passed, and I can concentrate. Little by little the symptoms are diminishing. I decide to try the vitamin IV once more. Again, I'm vomiting, unable to think. I'm so agitated. "You have to shut the IV off."

The supervisor has talked to Doctor Joe and my wish has been granted, but I'm not allowed plain IV fluid. There is to be no IV period. Worried and extremely thirsty, I sense it'll be a very long night.

**March 30**

Midnight. The supervisor has asked Bob and Dad, my security blankets, to leave. They were here to protect me from harm, to call the nurse if I needed help. What if I become foggy and confused again? Will I be able to call for help?

I have to ring the bell. Agitation wells up from the depths. Fogginess and confusion permeate my brain. I can't remember how the bell works. Momentarily, my mind clears, and I ring for the nurse.

What do I want? She's disappearing into the fog. What happened to the light in the room? I can't see her. Now she's back. She's asking questions. I'm paralyzed and can't answer.

After putting the blood pressure cuff on my arm and the stethoscope to my chest, she leaves the room. Unexpectedly, the room starts to clear, and I can move my hands a little. The nurse returns with a machine to check my blood sugar level. It's low, and she suggests this may be causing my problem. I ask her bring me the yams and wild rice Mom has cooked for me. If I try to eat, maybe the food will raise my blood sugar. With great difficulty, I move the spoon to my mouth.

The fog is settling in again. I need to use the washroom immediately. The nurse supports me for what seems like miles. I can barely sit up on the toilet. A violent pain crushes my back as I void, and I cry out as the flow of urine starts.

I lie awake, the waves of sickness in relentless pursuit of each other. Burning waves course through my bowel, alternately building and subsiding. I can't keep up with the thirst. The more I drink, the more I must struggle to the bathroom. Each visit brings more burning and excruciating pain to my back. I hang on to the sides of the toilet praying that I won't faint. Have my kidneys started to fail?

It's 7 a.m., and I've waited as long as I can. I phone Dad, crying. "Please come as soon as possible."

"I'll be there as soon as I can."

No one understands what's going on, including me. Why am I the sickest when Don's away? He would have stayed with me. No one can help me, and I can no longer help myself.

Doctor Joe is a gentle man. While sitting on the bed, he listens to my concerns. He has spoken with the allergist, and they have decided on the course of my treatment. I will work with the dietitian and drink the Formula recommended by Doctor Joan at the allergy clinic. Since Mom has explained my condition to Doctor Joan, I can ask for advice over the phone.

Doctor Joe's examination indicates I'm a healthy girl. However, he diplomatically suggests my severe thirst and numbness are related to the anxiety accompanying my illness. He would like the psychiatric team to make some recommendations. I respect him for his kind and gentle manner and I listen carefully to his words. From his perspective, these symptoms do mimic textbook anxiety. Although I know that's not my problem, I don't want to argue with him. He's trying to understand and has prescribed a reasonable avenue of treatment.

Curious about what the psyche team will decide, I agree to have the them examine me. I'm perfectly confident I can give the impression of someone without psychiatric problems. Besides, I can refuse any medication they may recommend. Expending my precious energy to appear sane is draining, but necessary. It's time for the medical community to fully acknowledge and validate all my symptoms.

## The Toxic Labyrinth

I can't believe my good fortune. Beth, the dietitian, has been in practice only three years, yet she's worked on a case with Doctor Joan. The condition of her patient, a woman who could not tolerate any food, including salt, seemed unbelievable at first. By the time Beth entered the picture, the woman had been admitted to the psychiatric unit. Working on that case has made her aware of how devastating allergies can be. Her former patient is now eating and leading a normal life. I shudder as she relates the story. At least I'm not that bad. Maybe there's hope for me yet.

Beth writes out the instructions. I must sip the Formula slowly, trying four cups throughout the day at first, so that my body gets used to it. Eventually I'll have to work up to six packets or twenty-four cups a day. I silently gag as we talk, remembering the vile smell of the Formula. Whatever is necessary to make myself well, I'll do.

Thankfully, I brought Formula and distilled water from home because it will be at least a week before the hospital can bring in a stock. Meanwhile, I can organize my own care rather than have the hospital send up premixed Formula. It's a small beginning, this attempt to control my recovery.

The jug on the bedside table reminds me of what lies ahead. Foul smelling and tasting, Formula will test my resolve. I know from my nursing experience the smell is caused by predigested proteins and carbohydrates. This knowledge won't make it taste any better. Well, I'd better get used to it. I pour the first drink and take a few sips. Immediately, my mouth dries. Gulping down a cup of distilled water, I continue.

The day is filled with the usual symptoms. Disturbing as they are, I've become used to these constant companions. The agitation of the past two days has disappeared. I'm still thirsty, but no longer compelled to drink eight cups of water an hour.

Dad notices my face flushes beet red and then becomes very pale. These color changes correspond with my symptom waves, the same effect as when I stopped the ranitidine. Why is Doctor Joe never here when these strange things happen?

It's evening. I look at the jug, the contents diminished by only one cup. Even though I've accomplished just a quarter of my goal, the Sahara Desert has laid claim to my mouth; my thirst is endless.

The TV is playing its usual role of distraction. Severe pains in my joints capture my attention. Suddenly, I can't blink my left eye, and the left side of my face is paralyzed. What's going on? I won't call the nurse; I'll wait for these symptoms to go away. The new sensation frightens me, not because it's more severe than the other symptoms, but it's different. I don't want to deal with the unfamiliar.

The feeling has returned to my face, followed by a slight burning in my chest and a generalized tingling. I wait, and finally, everything resolves.

I have fallen asleep for the first time in three nights. I awaken, later and smile, content that thirst is my only dilemma tonight. I drink two glasses of water and fall back to sleep.

**March 31**

As promised, the psychiatric team has arrived. The resident conducts the questioning, while the older doctor sits back in the chair, stroking his chin. I'm ready for them. Although I'm agitated and restless, I make my movements minimal so they don't pick up on this. I look straight into the doctor's eyes as he questions me. Yes, I was leading an extremely happy life until my illness struck. I was nursing when I wanted to and had the flexibility to take time off to travel with my boyfriend. I have a boyfriend who adores me and a supportive family. The doctor keeps inquiring about my happiness. Why does the medical world have such difficulty believing that a person can just be happy?

He asks me to calculate one hundred minus seven and to keep subtracting seven from the answer until he tells me to stop. I force myself to concentrate because it's important they conclude this is easy for me. No matter what my condition, I couldn't perform this task any faster. It's not a true test of mental stability, only a test of my mathematical skills.

I have him now. He wants to test my memory, which has always been my strong point. I think about people I know who don't have this ability and wonder whether they would be deemed mentally unstable if they couldn't remember eraser, pin, and book?

His eyes light up when I admit that my parents are divorced, a discovery about an imperfect childhood. However, I crush his speculation by stating my parents divorced when I was well into my twenties. Can he contact my mother? I tell him to be my guest. When he questions whether I'm depressed about my seven month illness, I ask in turn if he would be happy in the same situation. He smiles, all knowing. I'm not depressed, just exhausted by my inability to find an answer. Of course I'm angry about the months of testing, only to have one of the most vital pieces of information ignored until just recently. Depressed, no. Frustrated, yes. As they leave, the thought comes to me that a psychiatric team rarely confirms normal behavior. It'll be interesting to see if this team affirms my experience.

Doctor Joe sits on the bed and discusses the psychiatric evaluation. Of course, the team has recommended an anti-anxiety drug. He asks me for my opinion, and I'm elated he has sought my input rather than just writing a prescription.

"I want to try Formula for a month. If that course of action doesn't work, we can consider the other option." He nods in agreement.

After he leaves the room I smile inside. He's really listening to me and has advised me to remain in hospital to raise my confidence with the Formula. A dose of confidence, not drugs is something I very much need at this point. I vow again that my treatment will not involve drugs.

**CHAPTER 8**

# LOOKING INTO THE ABYSS

I look into the inviting blackness. There is an impulse within me that wants to succumb, but I crush it and fight on.

# The Toxic Labyrinth

## April 1

An early start to drinking Formula, day two. After deciding to drink at a rate of one third of a cup per hour, I pour the brew into a measuring cup so I can pace myself.

The pink bear nestles beside me on the bed. "This is a unique bear," Mom says. "She used to be a rather large grizzly bear, but she developed this allergy to people, and now there's nothing she can eat. As you can see, she is now a mere shadow of her former self. Still, she is alive and well, because she drank her Formula every day."

Mom is back perky as ever. I insisted she stay away from the hospital for at least a week, to rest, but two days away from the action was all she could stand. Just after visiting hours commenced, she breezed into the room carrying my pink bear, the blue quilt that has warmed me during each hospital visit, food from home, and another bag full of odds and ends she thought I couldn't do without.

When the day reaches the half time mark, I become braver and increase my drinking rate to one half of a cup per hour. This attempt makes my esophagus and stomach burn, and revives the nausea. Better stop drinking until my body settles.

My condition has greatly improved with the passing of the day. As the sun sets, I toast my consumption of four cups of Formula. The last drop disappears, swallowed with a sense of satisfaction.

## April 2

A more restful night, interrupted briefly by a severe headache and my relentless thirst.

My flu-like symptoms are more prominent today. Lifting the large jug of distilled water to mix my daily batch of Formula has exhausted me, and I lie on the bed to rest from the effort.

Almost half of my daily intake is consumed before noon, but my pride in this accomplishment is short lived. By one o'clock, the cramping in my stomach and esophagus is severe and my head is pounding. My body screams for water. Am I drinking too last? If I stop drinking for a few hours, will that help?

Symptoms bombarded my body all afternoon, and evening has not produced any relief. Although distracted by my symptoms, I try to visit with Mom. Why am I losing the sensation in my legs? An attack of nausea and retching abruptly changes the course of our conversation.

My blood sugar reading is very low, and Doctor Joe has refused my request for an IV. He has told the nurse, if I can't drink and tolerate four cups of Formula, my only other option is a feeding tube straight into the stomach. If I agree to the feeding tube, I will lose the hard won battle to manage my recovery. Right now, I can drink the exact concentration whenever I please. I'll try to stick it out for the night.

A quiet moment with Dad holding my hand. His touch conveys an understanding gained from a two-year battle with chronic fatigue. A new philosophy, molded from the desperation and destructiveness of that time, now directs his transition through life. He lives life to the fullest. Tonight he talks about that experience.

"Heather, I never thought I would get out of that bed. I lay there for months, sometimes too sick to raise my head, vowing to myself that if I recovered I would look at life differently. The vision that kept me going was the image of flying my plane, soaring over the ground, free from any ties on land."

His insight into the isolation and bleakness of a long term illness has drawn us closer. He speaks often of 'looking for the windows', the little victories which gave him hope. Now he encourages me to 'look for the windows', his words planting a small seed of hope that someday I may be able to live my life to the fullest, again.

# The Toxic Labyrinth

## April 3

Doctor Joe has recommended a day pass. Dad wheels my trusty hospital chariot to the car. Although I'm too weak to walk, I'm determined to spend some of Easter Sunday outside. We join the parade of cars down Robson Street. From the confinement of the car, I stare at the brightly lit windows. The street is a montage of businesses which invoke passersby with the aromas of international cuisine, tourist novelties, and stylish boutiques. Was it just last month I walked unaided past these same shops, a part of the energy of the street? Now even riding in the car seems to drain what little strength I can muster. The constant nausea and agitation are once again aimed at me, their preferred target. My voice rises in panic when I tell Dad to turn back. My Easter promenade will have to wait.

Wrapped in the security of my bedcovers, I engage in desultory conversation with Dad. As I look into his face, a surreal fog diminishes my vision. Dad, I hear what you're saying. Help me to form the answer. My hands are paralyzed, unable to attract your attention.

I must have blacked out. The nurse tightens the blood pressure cuff. Her voice mixes with Dad's forming a high pitched hum, but I can't make out their words.

"Heather?"

"Yes."

Dad seems relieved that I can talk again. He tells me I have been unconscious for almost an hour. The nurse has called the doctor to advise him about my abnormally low blood sugar reading.

The strange episode has passed, leaving me to deal with the onslaught of nausea and retching. Why am I so ill? Do I need sugar, salt? I shake violently. Cold seeps up from the tips of my extremities. Does the Easter Bunny bring good health? Apparently not.

Don is phoning from Africa. I grab the receiver. "Don, please come home," I beg in a voice filled with despair and panic. "I can't go through this without you any more."

188

"Heather, please give me the phone," Dad says.

"Don, there is no reason for you to come home. There are enough of us here to look after Heather. You can't do any more than we are already doing."

I'm angry because my life seems out of my control, and Dad is managing it. He doesn't comprehend my hopelessness. He's not the one with a spent body, alone in this hospital room, combating an endless series of mysterious challenges. Mom needs a break from nursing me and the daily hospital visits. Dad cannot be here all the time. I'm tired, too. Everyone seems to forget I'm the one who has been sick month after month, a captive in this body. Why do other people feel compelled to make decisions for me? I'm not a child. These days I can't always do things for myself, but I can think and I want Don home right now. Dad offers me the phone. I refuse to take it. Telling him to finish the conversation for me, I bury my head in the pillow and let the tears flow.

After the trauma of the day, a more tranquil aura has settled over me. Mom has agreed with Dad that Don's return would serve no purpose. Now that my symptoms have abated slightly, I can see the logic in their thinking.

The quiet of evening gives me time to develop my plan for introducing small amounts of food into my diet. Formula will give me the required nutrition until I can determine my safe foods. As I read the instructions from Doctor Joan, I realize this recovery process is more complex than other methods I have tried.

A tablespoon of boiled yams is my first attempt to reintroduce food. I have no idea what kind of reaction to expect. Since I'm experiencing symptoms constantly, how do I determine which symptoms are caused by the yams? If I make a record of my symptoms, before trying a food, maybe I can determine if the pattern differs once I've eaten. Formula calculations and food schedules race through my mind, a pleasant diversion from the constant preoccupation with symptoms.

## The Toxic Labyrinth

The nurse comes in to check on my progress with the Formula. She won't know I haven't been able to drink four cups. I've poured the remainder into the sink, pretending to have drunk it all. Satisfied, she leaves. I don't want the feeding tube. Control is important.

### April 4

Although it's early in the morning, I can't sleep. Struggling to sit on the edge of the bed, I wonder if I can summon the stamina to walk down the corridor. Keeping my Formula in the fridge means a trip down the corridor each time I require a refill.

As I step into the hall, a nurse insists she has to record my weight. I cringe as the scale indicates a loss of three more pounds.

Once again I'm surrounded by the elderly. Shuffling back to my room, I observe that each day is molding me further into this likeness. Near the nursing station, an old man sits strapped in a wheelchair, crying to everyone who passes to release him from his confinement. He has no choice, but to be controlled for his own safety. I clutch the jar containing my tenuous link to life and push through the door into my private space, the desolate voices of my elderly companions ringing in my ears. I place the jug on the bedside table and fall onto the bed to rest, my strength depleted.

Sufficiently, recovered from my venture to the kitchen, I begin my nutritional schedule. Sweet potatoes are today's food of choice and they taste marvelous compared to Formula. Even thinking about the taste of Formula makes me shudder.

Mom asks how I'm doing. What do I say? I can only cry. The bathroom is barely three feet away, but the effort to take a shower is more than I can manage even with her help.

Sitting on my bed and stroking my head she asks, "Heather, what's wrong?"

"I want a shower and I'm too weak to get out of bed."

"Well, you're not too weak for a bed bath."

A bed bath, it's come to this. I'm so glad Mom is bathing me;
I would rather die than allow a nurse to help me. There are limits to
the domination I'll allow this illness to have. The warm water soothes
my skin. Mom makes cheerful conversation as she braids my hair.
When she is finished I look in the mirror, satisfied with my new
image.

Knowing I'm too weak to sit in the chair, Mom changes the
bed linen, efficiently moving me from one side to the other. This
scene amuses me as no one except Mom has offered to change my
bed since my admission.

From the beginning, Mom has viewed my situation in the
most positive light, insisting that my progress will be similar to baby
steps, extremely slow at first, until finally I gain momentum. An
unenviable task, she has spent hours consoling me, pointing out the
smallest accomplishments. In her view, my sickness has taken time to
develop, so the time and effort expended for the cure will be
proportional.

After completing the ritual of comfort, she brings out the
progress chart she has designed. If I can focus on the positive, she
reasons, even my minor accomplishments will eventually lead to
good health. She's entitled the chart *Good Vibes List* or *Things That
Have Improved.*

I read the long list of symptoms that have disappeared in the
few days I have been drinking Formula: numbness in left hand,
confusion, insatiable thirst, waking up during the night, stomach pain
after drinking Formula, left flank pain, faintness, wrist pain, burning
in eyes, aching in legs, burning in chest, flu-like aches, constant
voiding, itching, hives on neck, and bruising. The IV is no longer
necessary and my extremities, although cold, are not nearly as cold as
they were.

Next, I focus my attention on the *Bad Vibes List* or *Things To
Get Rid Of:* right flank pain, weakness, burning in stomach, epigastric
burning, nausea, retching, and intermittent burning in left arm.

# The Toxic Labyrinth

Comparing the lists clearly illustrates the many assaults my body has been enduring and the immediate results from drinking the Formula. Baby steps, yes, I am moving with baby steps, although some major goals still remain. Can I accomplish these with increased intake of Formula and food?

Watching the clouds change patterns outside the window, I begin to realize the depth of sadness that has settled within me. The Easter weekend, a family time with special meals and traditions, has passed. It's hard to believe I haven't been able to work since the day I last administered pediatric medications in Memphis. How dramatically one's life can change overnight.

## April 5

Intermittent aches and pains have produced a drug-like but nervous sleep, which has left my body even weaker than usual this morning. Am I getting enough calories? Four cups of Formula is only three hundred calories, much fewer than the fifteen to eighteen hundred necessary to sustain me. I'll have to endeavor to drink more.

As Mom buttons my shirt, I look down at my jeans which now hang off my hips and project the image of a skateboarder striving to be one of the gang. What irony, I have spent my whole life trying to consume fewer calories. I love to eat and my body tends to show the results. Who is this strange creature, afraid of what the next trip to the scale might reveal?

Mom has prepared the back seat of the car as a bed. After I climb under the covers, I look back at the hospital entrance and watch an ambulance unloading its precious cargo. Each time I have been discharged, I have assumed it would be the last. This past year has been memorable in ways I would like to forget. Emergency rooms too numerous to count. Seven hospital admissions in seven months, seven years after my first bout with Crohn's disease. Is there a Biblical significance to my journey through this maze filled with detours and obscured sign posts? My last stay has given me time to reflect and

192

gain a sense of direction and control. Leaving this institution, I vow to set my own course. Although the path is not yet clear, my body, at its own pace, will reach my goal. Hopefully my luck has changed.

But ambivalence takes its turn as well. If I didn't recover after the other hospitalizations, what are my chances this time when I feel weaker than ever. It's hard to believe it is now April, and I'm no better. Is there a future for me? I'm not certain any more.

The only bedroom in the apartment is now my haven, specially designed to accommodate my confinement. Transformed into a hospital-like setting, the room offers all the conveniences at my bedside: tissues, straws for drinking, Formula boxes stacked in neat rows. Never one to miss a beat, Mom has even moved the bed closer to the bathroom. How lucky I am that she has been here for me one hundred percent, a key member of my aggressive support team of family and friends who still believe in what I am, and can be. As she helps me into bed, I realize how much the short ride home has exhausted my limited reserves.

I've decided to dilute the Formula to three quarters strength, a method suggested by Beth to increase my daily consumption. Almost eight cups before I close down this day. Despite some recurring symptoms, I'm satisfied with my progress and the increase in my nutritional elements. Even my temperature has finally returned to normal.

**April 6**

A good night's sleep, and I'm delighted. When I struggle to the kitchen to mix up my Formula—a task which gives me a measure of independence—I notice the burning in my esophagus and stomach has returned. I phone Doctor Joan for instructions and she cautions me against mixing Formula at the three quarters strength. Quickly, I revise my strategy.

The burning to my epigastric area has slowly disappeared, emphasizing the correctness of Doctor Joan's advice. No wonder I

# The Toxic Labyrinth

had such a violent reaction in March, when I first tried the Formula at four times this concentration.

Doctor John's receptionist escorts me immediately to one of the examining rooms so I can lie down. At least for this visit, I'm not retching and gagging throughout our conversation.

"Have you been back to Doctor A2?"

I feel guilty about not making an appointment. Doctor John has been supportive and caring, and I don't want to appear noncompliant.

"I'll make an appointment, immediately," I tell him.

I leave the office wondering what Doctor A2 can do for me. Now that I've set my own course of treatment, I really don't need his help, but feel obligated since Doctor John went to such lengths to arrange the first appointment.

My lunch consists of the two measly tablespoons of yams allotted for the day. How far in the future a meal of steak and potatoes appears when I'm introducing food in such minuscule amounts.

## April 7

Burning impulses migrate up and down the nerves in my back and invade my hands, rousing me into consciousness. The coldness, reaching from my feet into my knees, adds to my discomfort. What a gift it would be to sleep late each morning, to alleviate this never ending exhaustion and shorten the hours in the day. But today is successful. Twelve cups of Formula down the hatch. Quite an accomplishment for someone who is continually nauseated.

## April 8

Eyes open, staring at the ceiling, I attempt to fathom why I'm suddenly wide awake. Extreme thirst and agitation are vying for my attention. How can I describe this, except to say I hurt right into my brain. Too sick to move, I know if I lie still, this will pass like all the previous sessions.

All of my remaining symptoms, including a new addition to the roster, swelling on the roof of my mouth, greet me this morning. Even with the room temperature over ninety degrees, I shiver under the layers of quilts. Do I have the perseverance to leave the safety of my cocoon for the harshness of a trip to Doctor A2's office?

As Mom holds my arm, I shuffle, with hesitant steps, toward the car parked at the far end of the underground. She would bring the car closer, but setting little goals is important. Weak and nauseated, I sink into the back seat to conserve what negligible reserves remain for the next challenge.

Formula is my constant companion. Even in Doctor A2's office, I have to sip it continually. The daily schedule, a seventeen-hour routine of Formula and distilled water, is compulsory. Mom has gone back to the car for my water. My body craves water constantly, and the jug of distilled water accompanies me on all outings. The words of the psychiatrist flash through my mind, 'Drinking water is a sign of anxiety.' No, my constant thirst has nothing to do with anxiety. For some mysterious reason water and my path to wellness are inextricably connected.

"What can I do for you?" says Doctor A2, opening the conversation. Because I'm only here to be compliant, I really have no answer. He reports on his discussion with Doctor G3, who apparently had been quite bothered by the call. In the words of Doctor A2, they a gentlemanly chat about my condition. Or does he mean lack of condition?

It's obvious he is stringing out this session just long enough to work in his main point. With the pleasantries completed, he turns to Mom and asks if she has enough money to do whatever is necessary. Taken by surprise, she nods in agreement.

There are only two courses of action. The first is to arrange psychiatric help for me. And if that is not an acceptable avenue for her to pursue, she can, for ten thousand dollars, send me to the Mayo

# The Toxic Labyrinth

Clinic. He'll inform Doctor John of his findings. With that, he closes the file to signal the end of the visit.

Mom holds her tongue, but in a hostile voice thanks him for his advice. I'm furious. What is there to say? I've wasted time and precious energy only to be insulted. Too weak to express my disdain by storming out of his office, I must shuffle out, leaning heavily on Mom's arm. This visit has done nothing to bolster my confidence in the future.

Back in bed, scenes from the visit torment me. How many people as sick as I am, have been placed into institutions, and labeled as mentally ill? The thought is too disturbing and I push it from my mind. No one will do that to me. I will recover just to prove them all wrong.

The four tablespoons of yams have disappeared quickly. Normally, I roll the food around in my mouth and over my tongue to relish the taste. Today, symptoms override the fleeting pleasure of food, and nausea forces me to lie against the pillow while I contemplate my inability to distinguish a food reaction from my ongoing symptoms.

One always wants to place faith in something, to hope for a cure. I thought Formula would be the answer to my prayers, but it really has not met my expectations. Are they unrealistic? I thought a few cups of this magic mixture would be an instant cure. This has not been the case. My body is taking forever to build up to the mandatory twenty-four cups a day. Ingesting my daily intake of calories through a few tablespoons of food and twelve cups of Formula consumes my waking hours. Headaches and stomach aches are persistent companions of this miracle cure. Today is day ten of drinking Formula, and many of my symptoms have not yet resolved.

My sadness deepens, when I realize it may be many more months before I can return to work. What is the point in anticipating a future, if my attempts to date have met with failure? My vision is distorted by the overwhelming demands of my physical being. As much as it torments me to think about the future, it grieves me more to think about the past. The fun-loving, vivacious spirit has vanished, replaced by a frightened, emotionally devastated lump of diminishing flesh. I used to travel whenever the spirit moved me. Now, getting to the bathroom by myself is a major journey.

**April 11**

Well, all the questions remain. Why have my symptoms not completely vanished? There has been some improvement, but it's so slow. I have always been impatient, a person who expects results immediately.

Mom said something interesting today. 'Things happen for a reason. And at the time they are happening, you cannot perceive this reason. Maybe there is something wonderful that will come of this.' I guess we'll have to wait and see.

**April 12**

Bundled in blankets and a heavy jacket, I'm primed for an outing along the seawall in my rented wheelchair. I have agreed to this mode of transportation only because it gives me the means to leave the apartment.

Away from the hospital environment, I am quickly labeled 'disabled' by those who walk upright. These people who stride along the wall in perfect health avoid looking into my eyes, fearful of what they might see. They make me feel different, as if I'm purposely drawing attention to myself. How do people cope who are restricted to this life day after day? Objects always beyond reach. Accessibility denied. Every aspect of my life is becoming more of an effort.

I reflect on my experiences with this illness and the battery of tests which have not predicted any future treatment. My extensive list of symptoms mimic many of the illnesses that my children had experienced including asthma, arthritis, chronic fatigue, and cancer. Is there some meaning in this relationship? Forcing myself to eat, even when I'm not hungry has given me insight into the chronic nausea that accompanies cancer treatment. Many of my cancer children were confined to the hospital for months, their lives invaded by staff who poked, prodded, and gave them orders when their bodies craved only rest and solace.

Christmas Day was filled with sadness for those children who could not be at home with their families. I'm can empathize with their plight. This year I've been ill on New Years, my birthday, and Easter, each time hoping that the next holiday would be different. Only now am I beginning to realize how important those little extras mattered to my patients. How many times have I taken one of my children for an outing, such as this. The importance of that five minutes, for a child dying of cancer, cannot be defined.

Mom is trying her best, but the somewhat clumsy vehicle bumps along and the smallest impediment forces her to back up and try negotiating another route. The roughness of the street finally makes it impossible to ignore my nausea, and I terminate the outing.

When I was working, I used to wish for more hours in a day. The time off between shifts would fly by, leaving little time for contemplation or reflection. Now each day stretches into an endless path of nothingness, punctuated by the monotonous intake of Formula.

As usual, I'm looking at life outside the bedroom window and crying about my lack of progress. Mom sits on my bed and tries to refocus me. Everyday she reminds me that the cure will be slow and that I have to learn patience. Patience! Have I not been patient for seven months?

Mom takes out a file of papers, computer graphs and charts she has made from my daily records, and explains how they can illustrate my daily progress. Using them as a guide, I'll be able to judge my progress toward my goal of eighteen hundred calories of Formula and food.

The first paper is a chart that records Formula calories, the second is for food calories, and the third is a computerized version of the good and bad vibes charts, entitled *Heather's Daily Success Chart*. Each night before I go to bed, I can record my progress on these charts. The daily success chart will clearly show those symptoms that have been eliminated. Mom will make computer bar graphs from the entries on my Formula and food charts, so I can easily assess my progress. She has no intention of allowing me to sit and think about my illness. Even though it is ten years since she last taught school, her classroom techniques still surface at times like this. Refocusing my mind is key as far as she is concerned. A good thing for me, because in my present state, I definitely need to alter my perspective. And I have to admit, as I look at my progress in April, that more symptoms have disappeared.

**April 13**

Doctor Joe appears pleased with my progress when I show him my charts and graphs, proof of my determination. Eating yams, lamb, and sweet potatoes along with twelve cups of Formula gives me at least nine hundred calories. When I left the hospital, I was eating two foods and could manage just three cups of Formula. My voice relays my pride as I tell him of my accomplishments. He sits back in his chair, genuinely interested in what I am saying, and makes a few notes. When I step on the scale, his brow furrows with concern, and he comments on my further weight loss. Leaving his office more positive than usual, I congratulate myself. A two hour trip to the doctor! It has wiped me out, but I'm a long way from having to rely on Mom's assistance to bathe.

Later, I report my progress to Beth over the phone, and she suggests increasing the concentration of Formula to water, which will make my calorie intake easier. With my current mixing strategy, a daily intake of eighteen hundred calories would require twenty-four cups of Formula, as well as the extra water I require. She believes consuming such a large quantity of liquid will be too daunting a task.

# The Toxic Labyrinth

I sip the new concentration throughout evening, excited that I'm gaining ground. I've come a long way from my rudimentary beginnings.

**April 14**

Another early morning episode. My head is pounding, ready to burst. Thirst assails every pore and agitation joins the fray. These are not my usual combination of symptoms. Hopefully, reading will take my mind off this. I force myself, even though it's difficult to concentrate and focus my eyes.

Mom and I have decided that independent living will improve my outlook. Her one bedroom apartment, a necessary but cramped solution, has been home to four of us since December. Despite some symptoms from time to time, my charts illustrate progress each day and the elimination of many symptoms. It's time for the challenge of having my own space.

I have been excited about Don's arrival all week and even more excited about living in our own place. For some reason, on this day of his arrival, my excitement is overshadowed by a sluggish sickness. The familiar flu-like feeling lurks in the dark recesses of my body. When I push myself out of bed, my legs resist any rapid movement.

The small furnished suite, close to Mom's apartment, Doctor John's office, and a hospital, is as close to paradise as my current life allows. Mom has made all the arrangements and is helping me pack my few pitiful belongings. My life and possessions are still on hold at my apartment in Memphis.

The ride to my new home seems to take forever, despite its proximity to Mom's apartment. I emerge from the car and look at the flight of stairs before me. Only five steps, but today I might as well be looking at fifty.

The compact, sunny suite is a perfect abode for my convalescence, small enough for me to manage, and best of all, our own place. Don and I can throw our stuff wherever we want. Unfortunately, my happiness is overshadowed by the dizziness that is slowly inching its way into my day. Mom encourages me to lie down while she unloads the car.

I sink into the sofa, a heap of spent matter. Yesterday I was on top of the world, but today I have reverted to where I was weeks ago. Even the overwhelming cold is back. I would cry, but I mustn't cry on this special day. Although the smell of the lamb Mom has prepared for me is tantalizing, I'm so nauseated I have to force myself to eat.

Don has arrived and takes me into his arms. I sob into his shoulder. These days, his month in Nigeria seems like forever. He whispers everything will be all right now that he's home. Quietly he asks me about the last month; I trip over the words as I rush through the story. Even though we have spoken many times on the phone, he knows I need time to unleash my thoughts and feelings when he returns. As ill as I feel, he has raised my spirits.

In celebration of Don's return and our new apartment, I eat two more pieces of lamb.

## April 15

A quiet day spent drinking Formula, while Don recovers from his twenty-four hour flight. We laze around, luxuriating in our new digs, catching up on a month of news.

Exhausted from his flight, Don sleeps beside me. The print on the book before me swims in front of my eyes. The same pounding headache I experienced two nights ago has reappeared, accompanied by a feeling of agitation.

Have I drunk too much Formula? I perform a quick mental calculation and realize that, by 7 p.m., I have consumed three packages mixed at a much more concentrated strength than usual. Normally it takes me until midnight to drink an equal amount. Time to stop drinking and let my body readjust.

# The Toxic Labyrinth

I have tried to distract myself from the increasing symptoms, but my attention keeps returning to my current predicament. My tongue is swelling and this scares me. I keep swallowing to make the sensation go away, an approach that fails. Needing his reassurance to help me through this, I wake Don.

Finally, at 10 p.m. the nausea and insatiable thirst become all-consuming. There is not enough water in the world to quench my craving.

When it begins, the retching is violent, originating from deep within my body. Are my insides trying to come out through my face? Grabbing the sides of the toilet bowl tighter, I brace myself for the next violent wave. The progressive numbness in my hands is back, obliterating any sense of the cold, hard edge of the toilet. The back of my neck is on fire, and pain throbs through my flanks. A haze is slowly obliterating my vision. Don sits beside me on the floor, holding my hair and rubbing my back. I heave urgently, trying desperately to hold down what I have eaten during the day.

Thank God, the familiar and welcome shaking has arrived. I sit on the floor of the bathroom, trembling uncontrollably, while Don holds me in his arms.

## April 16

Day two hundred has dawned, ending a long night filled with sickness and thirst. Crying into the phone, I describe a day of setbacks to Mom.

"Mom, four cups seems to be my limit for Formula today. I'm nauseated and my tongue is swollen. When I try to eat, I'm retching within half an hour. I feel so sick."

"Just let your body rest. Drink water for a while. Don't worry about the Formula or about eating." Mom's voice has brought a measure of reason to this reversal in my progress.

I sit on the bathroom floor between bouts of retching. Most of my day has been spent here or in bed. I've been battling nausea, burning in the back of my neck, and extreme thirst. My stools are filled with blood. Can my body last through this? Don rubs my back and neck, trying to talk me through each spell. Thank God I have him. How do people manage who have to endure the trauma of chronic illness alone?

Sunset, and I'm happy to see this day come to an end. All that I have accomplished in the past two weeks has been destroyed in one day. Tomorrow I have to begin again by decreasing my Formula intake to four cups.

**April 17**

After a good night's sleep, just a few minor symptoms interfere with my day. My stool is almost normal, except for large pieces of mucous. Is all of this a good omen?

If I don't eat there is a danger I will lose all tolerance to food. I can't surrender this tiny bit of control and become a total care patient, completely dependent on Formula. Eating is my tie with normality, my passport to living in a conventional world.

During each visit, Doctor John has emphasized that I won't lose my ability to eat. In fact he says my body will quickly regain this function, even if I have to stop eating for a while. But I'm not that trusting any more. Too much has happened, making me wary of promises that may not materialize.

I've lost so much ground. Just over five hundred calories today no matter how hard I tried. The scale shows I've lost forty pounds since January. My body is ravenous one minute and nauseous the next. Too much food or Formula only makes it reject everything. I have to believe I'm doing the right thing. There is nothing more I can do.

# The Toxic Labyrinth

## April 18

Every day seems to revolve around the lack of calories and pushing my body further. Today I'll eat a small amount every two hours. The four hour rotation isn't working anyway. I have so many symptoms that identifying a food reaction is impossible.

Well, my plans for the day didn't work any better than anything else I've tried. The day was filled with pervasive cold and chills, nausea, and a myriad of other symptoms. Life has become one boring exercise of recording my progress or lack of it. Living at the survival level doesn't leave much time for lofty thoughts.

## April 19

I'm awake and completely frustrated. What can I do at 2:30 in the morning? Although I'm exhausted, I have awakened, agitated and unsettled. When I read, the page swims in front of my eyes, making it impossible to focus on the blurred letters.

I don't have a label. That's my problem. Under the current system, my problem eludes modern technology, so I can't be assigned a label. As a result, I will continually have to defend myself until a doctor can look inside my body and detect agitation and nausea.

The sun streams through the window. Usually I would welcome its warmth and light, but today I'm exhausted. Lately sleep is being rationed to me in small portions. Very early mornings follow fitful nights. Although I lie in bed for most of the day, my ongoing symptoms and low calorie intake leave me weak and tired.

Hooray! I have pushed myself up to eight hundred calories. Despite all that distracts me, I have held fast and reached a new goal, even managing to fight with the Louisiana State Nursing Board about the renewal of my license. One more baby step.

# Looking Into The Abyss

**April 20**

My fists pound into the pillow, punctuating each wave as the nausea and pressure inside my head build with each moment.

"Don, wake up. I need you to be awake with me. I'm scared." Even though Don can't make these spells go away, knowing he's awake and feeling his arms around me lessens the terror.

The morning brings the prospect of drinking Formula for the next seventeen hours. I look at the cup in my hand as the nausea rises into my throat. The smell assaults my senses, but if I'm to survive, there is no other avenue.

I'm too weak to make the twenty-pace trip to the fridge. Don brings me the afternoon allotment of Formula and sets it beside the bed. Suddenly, something inside me snaps.

"I don't want to be waited on. I've always been the caregiver. Lying in this bed like an old woman, depending on you to bring my Formula from the fridge will not be my role in life. I don't want to go on if this is my future." The rage inside me pours out, flooding into every corner of the room. I pick up a tissue box. Hurling it at the wall, brings an exhilaration I haven't experienced for a long time, and I continue throwing any object within my grasp.

Don stands in stunned silence for a moment, then walks over and takes my hands. "Heather, your dependence on me is for a very short time. Some day our roles may be reversed. You may have to look after me in the same way I am looking after you right now. We don't know what changes will come into our lives over the years. When two people love each other, they don't have roles, they just fulfill each others needs, one day at a time."

Deep down I know he's right, but the urge to rebel remains strong. Drinking Formula is not a matter of choice. I don't have the option of missing even one day. Unlike other types of therapy, which one can occasionally skip, my seventeen hour shift is etched in stone.

# The Toxic Labyrinth

## April 21

I stumble against Don while we silently pace around the small living room. The ringing in my ears makes conversation impossible. As weak as I am, the early morning symptoms exploding through my body are so overwhelming, I can't remain in bed.

A visit to Doctor John. He assures me my weight loss is not yet at a critical point. and encourages me to keep making the effort. Even though he doesn't know what is wrong with me, the fact that he understands I need his reassurance is comforting. His kindness and compassion spur me on.

A welcome present at the end of the day, my symptoms are somewhat resolved. The waves of illness have diminished, leaving me tired and less agitated.

## April 22

Funny how the morning seems brighter, more friendly after an undisturbed sleep. Don and I sift through the articles on food intolerance from Internet. I make many phone calls, each time requesting information that might give us some direction. Our pool of data indicates help is out there, if we can only locate it. There is an allergy clinic in Washington, just a short drive from Vancouver, and I make an appointment for May.

The afternoon light plays on the ocean swells while Don and I sit on the beach, the warmth of the sun bathing our bodies. I sip my Formula from a covered cup, protecting my lifeline from the sand with plastic wrap. On days such as this, I can retreat from the abyss and reaffirm my determination to meet the challenge that has been thrust upon me.

## April 23

The eggs, their vivid colors proclaiming the ancient ritual that is part of my heritage, are nestled in their display boxes. Don has insisted we attend the show of Ukrainian Easter eggs at the art gallery. Usually he teases me about my love of crafts and my ever-increasing collection of handicrafts. Today he encourages my interest, however fleeting, in something other than my illness. He worries I am losing interest in those activities I love the best.

Watching the traffic as it hustles by, I sit on a bench at the bus stop waiting for Don to return with the car. The familiar weakness is slowly seeping into my body, and I know it's time to return home.

A little nap and something to eat should give me the strength to attend the Grace's shower. Thankful the agitation that has plagued me for days has diminished, I close my eyes and luxuriate in an short afternoon nap.

Grace is delighted I am well enough to attend her shower. Who can I sit beside? A chair next to someone I know will set my mind at ease. Conversation will not be difficult with an old friend. If I become disoriented, my knowledge of times and places will help to hide any confusion.

The group is talking about Cynthia, a friend we all knew from university. While traveling for business, she came down with a slight flu. After an evening of socializing, she went for a run in the morning before catching her flight. The attendants, thinking she was asleep, tried to rouse her when the plane landed and discovered that she had died enroute. The story sends waves of terror through me. Will this be my fate? My problems began with flu-like symptoms.

I've stayed an acceptable amount of time, thirty-five minutes. As she sees me to the door, Grace mentions that I look unwell. Don is waiting in the car, as he insisted on remaining close at hand in case I needed anything.

A hot bath will relieve the constant cold permeating to the very core of my soul. Don draws the bath. Wanting to add something

# The Toxic Labyrinth

special to the water, I take the bottle of aromatherapy oil from the shelf and remove the cap. The scent permeates the bathroom, and my head reels in response to its pungent odor. I quickly replace the cap and climb into an unadulterated bath.

## April 24

Walking slowly along the beach with Don, I marvel at the way the ocean revitalizes me. For some reason, my body has developed an affinity for water.

We stand in front of the ice cream store. I can only watch as Don runs his tongue over the creamy mound topping the cone. How can I deprive this man, my support through all this emotional devastation in our lives, of so simple an indulgence? The smell of the ice cream invades my senses, reminding me of pleasures past. Mentally, I savor each lick right down to the last crunch until the stem of the cone passes into oblivion.

## April 25

I have spoken with Doctor Joan on the phone, now it's time to meet in person. As I put on my shoes in preparation, the waves of nausea and other symptoms make me uncertain about expending the effort. What more can she possibly do for me?

Doctor Joan is elegant, her faint accent adding mystery and allure. This woman, a brilliant nutritionist and immunologist, introduced me to Formula, the tenuous thread connecting me to the world. In the beginning, I had believed that Formula was a quick fix, and in just a few days, I would feel amazingly better. Now as I listen to her quiet consultation, I begin to realize the time commitment that getting well will demand.

The three of us sit in her cramped office, hanging on each word. Doctor Joan talks about introducing food more slowly, about letting my symptoms clear completely before I try to eat again. The room spins around me, but my pride determines that my demeanor must give the appearance of coping. Besides, I can't let her think I'm unable to follow orders, or give her any reason to abandon my cause. On our way out, we stop at the receptionist's desk to pick up the names of other women who are on Formula. Mom is certain that contacting these women will make me feel less isolated. We'll see.

**April 26**

The laser light show at the Planetarium pierces my brain. Closing my eyes, I attempt to hang on. Don asks so little of me, the least I can do is stay until the end. On our way to the car, I collapse on the steps. Don scoops me into his arms and carries me to the parking lot.

Don and I play cards with Dad. The impact of the laser show has diminished, and the fog which has enveloped my brain all day is lifting. Even the ringing in my ears has disappeared. I concentrate on the game, noting that the card markings are distinct.

**April 27**

Each day I get closer to consuming nine hundred calories of Formula. No food for me these days. Doctor Joan has instructed me to clear my symptoms first.

Don pushes the wheelchair while I walk unaided down the hill. I don't require my chariot, not today. How long has it been since I could manage such a feat? An eternity. Although it's just a little hill, the accomplishment is all mine.

The afternoon sun warms my soul. Our pale white limbs provide a stark contrast to the green blanket. Two colorless bodies soak in the light, hoping to repair the ravages of winter. A soft breeze ripples the water in the pond below. The sound of his voice flows around us, as Don reads aloud from a novel.

## The Toxic Labyrinth

The sun has renewed my vitality. Up and down the stairs to the laundry in our apartment: washing, drying, folding. Don can hardly believe my energy tonight.

I have phoned Debra, a member of the Formula support group, who informs me she has been on Formula for over a year with no signs of improvement. Why did I phone? This is not a story I need to hear right now.

The paper in front of me fills with words of encouragement. I am writing Dad's cousin, Lois, who has been ill for three years. She can eat very little and has been bedridden for some time. Much of what she is experiencing sounds familiar. Although I am not certain I am the best person to give her hope, perhaps we can support one another.

### April 28

Doctor John is pleased with my progress. I'm feeling much better today and it shows. I inform him about my visit with Doctor Joan, and that I'm not eating so my symptoms will clear.

Another day in the sun at the park. Don and I lie on a blanket laughing and cuddling. It's wonderful to talk about something other than my illness.

## CHAPTER 9

# THE WELL

**I can only compare my ordeal to this. I feel as though I have been at the bottom of a well, wet and cold for a very long time.**

## The Toxic Labyrinth

**May 1**

Don is off to Memphis to pack and move our belongings from the apartment. How long our lives will remain in limbo is still undetermined. Most of our possessions will be stored in Memphis, until we are able to devise future plans.

When I moved from contract to contract, I was used to living out of a suitcase. The decision was a conscious one, made to enjoy a variety of different jobs and the spontaneity of travel. Although I am still living out of a suitcase, my possessions residing in various cities and storage lockers, the feeling is much different. Bits and pieces of my life are scattered about. Nothing is where it should be.

Good news on the home front. I have climbed back to nine hundred calories today. Cold still holds my body captive, but most of the other symptoms have disappeared. Doctor Joan's plan appears to be working.

**May 2**

What is happening? Why do I always have problems when Don leaves? I haven't had early morning symptoms for days. Am I just anxious because Don is not with me? No, I have these same symptoms when he is with me. They will pass in a few hours, if I am patient.

I have managed the short walk from the apartment to the lab by myself. Standing in lobby of the medical building, I contemplate the return journey.

"Hi, Heather," the friendly voice calls.

The greeting comes from an acquaintance I haven't seen since university days. I don't want to meet people who knew me when I was fun-loving and energetic, not when I look like I do today. But there is no escaping this encounter. Feeling the faint stirrings of nausea, I search for some means of support, even a post will do, to

212

prop me up during this meeting and I play out the charade that everything in my life is fine.

Even though the visit has depleted my limited reserves, it's important to my self esteem to walk the three blocks home. I push myself to take a few steps, only to return to the security of the lobby when that attempt fails. One more try. Back to the lobby again. Finally, admitting that I am not going to meet this challenge, I phone for a cab.

I look down at my hands. It seems today is ending the same way it started with swollen hands. A new symptom, just what I need.

## May 3

The mixture of overpowering and harsh odors increase my nausea as I walk down the drugstore aisle to buy more Formula. Why have I never noticed this until now? I urge Mom to walk quickly to the counter so we can transact our business and leave.

Formula is saving my life, but at price of one thousand dollars a month. Mom rationalizes the cost. How else am spending money? She's right: no dinners out, no new clothes, no flowers, nothing, except days of drinking Formula. In order to save my life, I have given up all the things which used to give me pleasure. There is no softness to my existence now, only the harsh reality of survival.

When Mom backs the car out of the parking space, a sharp scraping sound rises above the sound of the engine. It appears a souvenir piece from the concrete post will accompany us back home. Looking at the large gouge stripped of paint, over the right front wheel, Mom laughs, "Heather, the car is old. This scrape balances some of the damage on the other side. Besides, it's so infinitesimal in the scheme of our lives right now."

# The Toxic Labyrinth

**May 4**

My nausea and restlessness have escalated steadily the last few days, making it necessary to call Doctor Joan. Like me, she is worried about my calorie intake, and urges me to increase my daily consumption of Formula. It's my only form of nutrition until I can begin eating again.

Increasing the Formula has made me even worse. Why do I always have problems when everyone is away? Don will be home by Friday, but that seems like an eternity in my life these days. Phoning from a conference in Whistler, Mom listens to my plight and warns I may be drinking at too rapid a rate, and my body may not ready. Why can't I handle an increase of one eighth of a cup per hour?

Jane has come to visit for the evening. While she talks about her day at work, my mind wanders from the conversation to the agitation and uncertainty in my body. I'm having difficulty talking. Finally, I stop drinking Formula. I'm too ill.

**May 5**

Another early morning awakening. Afraid to be alone, I concentrate on remembering how to dial the phone. When my confusion temporarily lifts, I dial Bob's number. After the answering machine quips a cheerful greeting, I leave a message, hoping that Bob will be home soon. Regardless of the circumstances, I can depend on Bob during times of crisis. Over the years he has brought a lot of warmth and goodness into my life. A short time later, Bob arrives at my door, and the comfort and reassurance of his presence allays my fears for the moment.

Bob has brought me to the welfare office in my wheelchair. Are there any more defeats remaining on my journey to nowhere? As I wait to be processed, I become one of the blank faces sitting along the wall. Who are we? Ordinary people unlucky enough to be struck down in our transit though life.

With each passing minute, the interview is becoming more degrading. I'm not allowed to have any cash or own any valuable possessions, not even a car. How does someone escape the clutches of welfare, if the guideline for financial assistance is destitution? What little independence and self respect I still have is slowly eroding, like Chinese water torture. I don't want to depend solely on Mom and Don for financial assistance, but I can't quite bring myself to enter the government system.

Don's voice fails to soothe me. He has been calling three times a day from Memphis. I want him here with me, not hundreds of miles away. Why does our time together have to be manipulated by my illness?

**May 6**

Another day of headache and constant thirst. I can't seem to drink enough Formula, and I'm under nine hundred calories again.

Don holds me, soothing my fears. Why do I go from one crisis to the next, always emotionally devastated by my inability to cope? I never used to cry. I didn't have time for such nonsense.

My friend, Rita, who is looking for a job in Vancouver, is coming to stay with me. Mom will be away for two weeks, and Don is returning to Africa. One minute I'm well enough to be on my own and the next I'm dependent on live-in care.

**May 7**

My body is controlling my life as usual. For some reason, my condition has been declining lately. Grace's wedding is today, an event I have anticipated for months. Don has offered to take me in the wheelchair, but I'm too ill to manage, even with assistance. If I did

## The Toxic Labyrinth

feel well enough to attend, I have too much pride to allow friends, whom I have not seen recently, to see me surrounded by the trappings of my chronic illness.

As I sit by the window, the bright day is a painful reminder of the missed invitation to laughter and good times. My only diversion is TV. I don't want to watch TV, this reminder of my incarceration.

"Heather, there will be something to replace this wedding. You'll see," Don says trying to console me.

"There is nothing that can replace the time I've lost since last September. It's gone. I can never have it back. Soon it will be summer, and I will miss that, too."

"It's always summer some place in the world. When you are better, I will take you to where it is summer."

**May 9**

Watching Don's tall frame settle into the back seat of the taxi reminds me that another month has come and gone. I don't know what is worse—the symptoms that continue their constant assault, or the emptiness when he leaves.

I have not eaten for two weeks, a strategy that has made little difference. If my problem is a simple food allergy, then why am I not improving when I don't eat?

Today I will try turnip, a food that is low on the allergy scale. Since I have seldom eaten this food, my body hasn't had the opportunity to create antibodies against it. What if I try one tablespoon just as a test? This vegetable has never been a favorite food, but today it's gourmet fare. Savoring the bouquet and biting flavor, I roll the small helping around in my mouth, as long as I can, before swallowing.

Until I was compelled to forego food, I never realized how much our society revolves around eating. My only entertainment is TV, a medium dominated by advertisements for food in some form:

packaged, fresh, restaurant meals. Each day I'm bombarded by images of something I cannot have, no matter how accessible.

When Don cooks a meal, he doesn't want to eat in front of me, but I insist. I want to eat vicariously through his meals, to take part in the activity, to steep myself in the aroma of steak, baked potato with bacon bits, butter, and sour cream. Inside, I'm angry that he can eat, yet I'm compelled to watch, fascinated by what I'm denied.

However, I'm not totally genial about this scenario. Don relishes foods loaded with fat and cholesterol which, I caution, are taking a toll on his health. What has happened to me was unexpected. I appeal to his sense of fair play, emphasizing that it's easy for him to encourage me to drink my Formula, while he eats up a fatty storm. Realistically, I know I would say nothing, if I could eat what he is eating. After all, I was a hundred and sixty pounds back in September, a weight I attained through a less than healthy diet.

The buzz of the intercom punctures my thoughts.

"Yes."

"Delivery for Heather Millar."

Who would be sending me a parcel? I punch the access button.

"Hi, my flight was delayed. You have me for one more night."

Who cares about eating habits.

**May 10**

Rita, my new caretaker, and I exchange news. She has just returned from smoking a cigarette on the balcony, and although I'm sitting across the room, the traces of cigarette smoke from her clothes are making me nauseous. I've always had a heightened sense of smell, but never to this extent. So many odors seem to bother me these days: laundry detergent, cleaning products, pepper, even cooking odors.

# The Toxic Labyrinth

## May 11

Why does this office confuse and disorient me? As I speak with Doctor Joan, I have trouble looking into her eyes. For some time, I've found it impossible to fix my gaze on an object or person for any period of time. Even before my illness, I would lose my concentration when driving on the interstate after work or during a long trip.

"I can't seem to bring my intake of Formula up to nine hundred calories without crashing below that level a few days later."

"Heather, you have no other options." I know Doctor Joan is right, but my body is holding me back.

The scale registers a ten-pound weight loss since I last saw her in April. I read the concern in Doctor Joan's face and hear the anxiety in her voice. This reinforces my fear about lack of calories and poor nutrition. In desperation, I start to cry, even though I realize she is just encouraging me to go on, not reprimanding me. Still, I feel like a bad child unable to meet mother's demands. Why won't my body cooperate? I want so much to comply with Doctor Joan's directions, especially since she is the first person to devise a solution for me. She is keeping me alive.

In the waiting room, I compose myself before my appointment with Doctor Joe. If he suspects things are not going well, he may prescribe anti-depressants. I don't have to take them, but I don't want that treatment on my file. Doctor Joe is confident I will reach my goal. He counsels me to prepare for further weight loss before this happens. Apparently, my weight will stabilize when I can consistently consume a minimum of nine hundred calories. His remarks relax my fears, and I leave determined to try again.

## May 12

The symptoms that have persisted for days have continued throughout the night and remain with me this morning. Burning in my

218

eyes, chest, back, and mouth. Cramping in my hands and feet. Numbness in my face. Hip bones that ache with the cold even though the temperature in my room is over ninety degrees. The only improvement, the roof of my mouth is not swollen.

Doctor John offers his usual brand of encouragement. Even though he knows I want independence, he discusses the possibility of TPN (total parental nutrition) as a last resort. Such treatment would mean returning to the hospital and feeding through an IV that goes straight into the heart. I would have to be on my death bed before allowing this. Some of my cancer children had to live this way, and while there is the chance of infection, the biggest nightmare is that drugs are administered through this avenue into the body. If the nurse is not proficient, medication or IV fluids can be administered too quickly, inducing negative reactions in the patient. The effect of the vitamin IV is still fresh in my memory.

Doctor John also talks about anorexia. Although he does not think I'm anorexic, my body is in a similar state because of my nutritional deficiencies. Will I agree to see a physician who can deal with the physical aspects of this condition? I have no difficulty with his suggestion, since I'm eager to gain any information on nutrition.

Rita had read the tarot cards for Don before he left for Nigeria. The cards had revealed that Don would receive an important message at work. We'll see about that. At the time, I was afraid to see what the cards held for me. Today my curiosity is peaked. Rita lays out the cards, and I watch with fascination as she turns up each prediction. Will the death card appear?

"According to the cards, your future holds the promise of money, new employment, and new interests especially in spiritual matters. However, the path to attainment is marked by uncertainty, crises, and wasted energy. In the last six months the factors of hope, courage, inspiration, and unselfish aid have become part of your experience.

# The Toxic Labyrinth

"The future may hold marriage, material happiness, and major achievements, but your current fears revolve around things lost and the uncertainty of new environments and horizons to come. The last card, the chariot, is a sign for those who will achieve greatness.

"Heather, all your cards are major cards. I wish my future held such promise," Rita says.

Will my future include conquest, success, and triumph over money difficulties and ill health? There are no guarantees in the cards, nevertheless, I want so much to believe.

Mom has phoned me twice a day from Los Angeles. Her reassurance acts like a drug and keeps me going.

"I looked in the mirror today. There is no more fat on my back. Every single bone in my spine is showing," I tell her.

"If it bothers you to look in the mirror, don't look in the mirror. You should only concentrate on one thing, drinking Formula. Right now you can't worry about anything else." Practical as usual, Mom has cut right to the heart of the matter.

"Heather, I don't want to you try any more food until I return. Right now, the little food you are eating makes no difference to your calorie intake, instead it seems to make you sick."

"I'm so exhausted. I can't drink for seventeen hours a day. I want to try a feeding tube so that I can rest for a few days."

"You know best, Heather. This is the second time you've had to start at three hundred calories. Don't increase the amount of Formula by more than five percent each day. I think you're trying to increase your rate too quickly."

**May 13**

"Doctor John, my symptoms keep me awake at night and I'm too exhausted to drink Formula for seventeen hours a day. Can you possibly arrange for me to have a feeding tube?" Although this is an undesirable method of intake, I have to do something to keep going.

If I can be fed through the night, that will provide a calorie intake for twenty-four hours, instead of just seventeen. I hang up the phone, grateful that Doctor John has listened to me and will make the necessary arrangements.

What I thought would be easy has turned into a bureaucratic nightmare. The head nurse at the hospital will only give me a gravity drip bag and I don't want this. A gravity drip bag requires a full-time nurse to regulate the flow. I want a feeding pump, so that the flow of Formula is calculated and delivered automatically by the computerized pump. The head nurse won't agree to put the tube down unless I am on a special program through the hospital, and has no further suggestions. To conclude our conversation, she informs me I have no business asking emergency to perform this service. The staff are too busy to accommodate me.

Community Health can't assist me unless I'm on home care after a hospital discharge. In addition, I need a prescription in order to obtain a feeding pump from them.

Several more calls bring no satisfaction. But I am determined to find a solution. Through my nursing experience in the United States, I know I can go across the border and set up my own system. If it is necessary, I will go to these lengths. My last call is to a medical supply company. Feeding pump? No problem. All I need is money.

Doctor John has called a second time to check on my progress. He offers to put the tube down, but suggests one of my nursing friends would be a better choice. This procedure is part of their daily routine. These words corroborate my decision; he is on my side.

Although my eyes tear and I gag continuously throughout the procedure, Melodie slips the tube down my throat with practiced efficiency. The loathsome process is difficult to perform on a stranger, let alone a friend. Since Melodie has taken the time to do this for me, I would like to visit, but the tube makes this impossible.

# The Toxic Labyrinth

My throat is raw and painful, and the slightest movement of my head makes me gag.

**May 14**

Unfortunately, the feeding tube cannot accomplish its main purpose. My body won't adapt to the intake of Formula over a twenty-four hour period. This constant intake of Formula increases the symptoms beyond a bearable level. I guess my body needs a rest during the night. Even if twenty-four hour feeding was a possibility, I would have to sleep sitting up, because the tube makes me choke. However, I can set the tube to run first thing in the morning, a strategy which allows me the chance to sleep in. I haven't achieved my whole goal, but these days, half a goal is acceptable.

Rita and I calculate the increase of Formula. Starting with one third of a cup per hour, I will increase my daily rate by one teaspoon per hour. Every three days, I will drink at the same rate, permitting my body to adapt to that level. My body won't allow me to push it any faster, and I try not to think about my initial intake of three hundred calories.

Click, click, click around the TV channels. Commercials about diet plans, talk shows about weight loss fill the afternoon programming schedule. Is there no other topic of concern in this universe? Was it just last year I fretted about my weight problem? Dieting for two days, then quickly reverting to former eating habits. When we lived in Memphis, Don would tease me that I was on the Elvis Presley diet.

Maybe my tendency to be overweight has its merits. All through this ordeal my stomach has retained some fat, while the rest of me wastes away. Pauncherelli, as Don has named this souvenir of former excesses, lives on, but in a much reduced state. This final reserve is my marker. When it is depleted, I know all is lost.

## May 15

The balls of wool in variegated shades of blue spill across the blanket. My love of crafts does not extend to proficiency in knitting. Who has time for this when there are parties, fun, and friends? But times have changed. When I pick up the needles to knit a stitch, my fingers and arms lose energy with this simple movement. Knit ten stitches; stop to rest. How much my life has shifted to the ways of the elderly.

Although the feeding tube is painful, it provides an opportunity for me to rest. How can anorexics prefer this option to eating? But should I be so judgmental? Maybe their bodies are resistant to food, just like mine. Before now, I have never looked at anorexia from that viewpoint.

## May 16

I'm gaining ground almost imperceptibly, a progress marked only by small increases in Formula intake. Each day has become a never-ending march toward evening and is made more endurable through the oblivion of the naps guaranteed by the feeding tube.

I stare at my face in the hand mirror. Acne. Even as a teenager, I didn't have acne. How does my body have the energy to create pimples? There must be more useful tasks for it to perform with the limited nutrition it receives.

Nursing myself at home is a strange, but comfortable concept. My children who had to be tube fed detested being confined to the hospital. How much more soothing it is to be at home in one's own space, surrounded by the familiar.

Doctor Joan has warned me not to spend time in public places. My immune system is suppressed, and I can easily catch a virus. Rita has a cold, and my nose has started to run. How do I blow it without pushing out the feeding tube? What are my chances of shaking off this virus? Can anything more happen to me?

**May 18**

Don is calling from Nigeria. After typing my story onto the Internet, he has had several responses from people recommending a place called The Clinic. I cry at the thought. Not a clinic. No more hospitals. What have medical institutions done for me so far? Don is resolute and instructs me to contact Kathy, one of the correspondents. Thinking about Don's words gives me pause. Is it just coincidence or did the tarot cards reveal the future? Messages from the Internet. Voices giving us hope.

Kathy relates a horror story of exposure to pesticides that has led to a fifteen-year illness. Now there are many places she can't go, things she can't do, foods she can't eat, and chemicals she can't tolerate. These intolerances prevent her from carrying on a normal life. Although she has an interesting story to tell, my problem is food allergies. I don't have any problem with carpets, shampoos, perfumes, plastics, pesticides, and all the other items she lists.

I talk to Doctor Joan once a week, so she can record my progress and encourage me to continue my feeding program. Because my situation is critical and must be monitored closely, she insists I also keep in touch with Doctor John.

**May 19**

If nothing else, my curiosity is aroused, and I have requested information from The Clinic. Experience has taught me to be cautious and to check the credentials of doctors I might consider as part of my recovery process.

With a feeding tube up my nose, attending to my personal needs is not easy. Aside from the fact that it is connected to my face with a massive wad of tape, there is still room for error. The feeding pump is attached to a pole, which tends to catch on the rug. When rug and pole come into contact, I trip. As I fall forward, the tube jerks and swings making me gag. There must be a comedy routine inherent in this predicament.

## May 20

The tube is out. Although my throat is raw, the tube has served its purpose by giving me a week of rest.

Appointments with two professionals who will assist me psychologically mark another advance in maintaining control over my recovery. Mom and Rhonda have subtly suggested that counseling from someone other than a family member would help me through this crisis and my emotional shoals.

Steve, a counselor, who had advised me when my greatest decision revolved around employment changes, has agreed to speak with me over the phone, because I'm too weak to make an office visit. While he listens intently, I pour out my story. We speak of many things, and toward the end of our conversation, he makes an interesting comment.

"Heather, you shouldn't be alone. Other people create an energy flow your body lacks in times of chronic illness, an energy they can transfer to you." Maybe it's time to change my living arrangements. I spend entirely too much time by myself.

Daryl and I speak often. During our discussions, he has mentioned several times that western medicine may not have all the answers, an interesting remark from a medical researcher. He has given me the number of his sister, Akash, whom I haven't seen since we nursed together a number of years ago. I'm not clear what she can offer. Some method of meditation, I gather from his description. I have made an appointment with her, anything to distract me from endless days of nothingness.

# The Toxic Labyrinth

I turn on the tape recorder. "I can only compare my illness to this. It is as though I have been at the bottom of a well, wet and cold for a very long time. When I first tumbled into the well, I suffered only a few minor bruises. I was still strong and just needed a rope to help me scale the cold and slimy sides. My friends and family had seen me fall and gathered around the top of the well. Offering words of encouragement, they peered down to see if I was all right.

"But the walls were too slippery for me to climb out unassisted, no matter how much encouragement I received. After a time, my strength waned leaving me cold and hungry. Finally, after many days had passed, help arrived when someone threw me a rope, so I could climb out of the frigid and dark place. Whatever strength remained was minimal. Could I find the energy to climb out. My aching arms unsteadily gripped the rope, and ever so slowly I climbed up the slippery sides. When I could almost grab the top of the well, I paused for a second to look back to where I had been. The sight reminded me of such a traumatic and terrible time that I froze with fear. That momentary paralysis prevented me from making it to the top, even though I was so close."

**May 22**

On her return, Mom insisted that I move back with her, so she will be able to care for me without commuting between the two apartments. Although Rita has been an excellent care giver, she is starting a new job and will be away for much of the day.

I look out the window at the bridge, this scene so much a part of my being. How many days have I watched the cars make flickering patterns on the wall as they pass through the sun's rays?

Steve is right. Living at Mom's creates an energy in me. People are moving about, are doing things. Mom scurries in and out, never leaving me long enough to brood about what is ahead.

**May 24**

Doctor Joan has assured me that once my symptoms have disappeared completely, and I reintroduce food, my tolerance will gradually return. Her support is welcome. Continual reassurance has become one of the cornerstones of my recovery.

Dad has sent my great, great grandmother's Bible by special delivery. As I hold this treasure in my hands, I think of Steve's suggestion to discover my inner soul. What better way than through this possession of a powerful woman who was in touch with her spiritual self. Can she help me find peace? The page is open to the Psalms, passages Steve has suggested I read to give me hope. My great, great grandmother has written thoughts and notes on many pages of this Book, used as her daily guide. If I memorize some of the Psalms, maybe they will bring me peace at times when I need to concentrate on something other than my symptoms.

**May 25**

I haven't awakened at night for a long time. The agitation has pushed me into consciousness. My eyes light on the Bible beside me, but I'm too sick to read. The words of Psalm Twenty-three run through my head. If I repeat this passage, will it give me strength? Even if the Psalm is the one most often recited at funerals, it's the only one I know by heart. "The Lord is my Shepherd . . ."

Although the thermostat reads over ninety degrees and the sun is shining across my bed, I am freezing and unwell. Carol is coming to visit this afternoon. How can I manage to be sociable?

Akash has arrived to give me my first session, complete with a folding treatment table and her right arm in a cast. No matter what it involves, the session will provide a distraction from the interminable time in this cell. I can read for only short periods, and my knitting has progressed to the point where I can complete a row

# The Toxic Labyrinth

before having to rest. Despite these diversions, there are many more hours to fill. Yes, Akash is a welcome sight. Rhonda will be proud of my daring departure into the world of alternative medicine.

I was expecting a massage, but instead Akash is explaining a process called Healing Touch. Her chocolate brown eyes and dark hair add to the mystery, as she discusses chakras, energy fields, and the placing of hands over the body. What is this hocus-pocus? While she spins a crystal above my chest, she explains to Mom why the crystal is moving in certain directions. We're into the twilight zone now, but I don't care. One less hour to fill on my own.

I close my eyes while Akash moves her hands in a sweeping motion six inches from my body. Even though the force of this action creates an intense heat, which moves violently from my feet to my head, I refrain from stopping her. My mind takes its own course, repeating over and over, "I have to get better.".

Mom's voice cuts into my consciousness. Akash is teaching her about the chakras. Holding the crystal above my body, Mom remarks that it moves without her assistance. Like me she is very practical and is trying to fathom the energy forces affecting the crystal.

I'm sitting up laughing and talking with Carol, my body warmer, more relaxed. I can even focus on her face, without having to avert my gaze every few seconds. My whole being has responded to the potent forces of Healing Touch. What strange power resides in Akash's hands? Now that I have more control over making myself well, what other secrets will I discover?

## May 26

Two weeks since I was last outside. Closing my eyes and throwing back my head, I invite the sun to wash over my face. Doug pushes the wheelchair while Mom and I decide which route to take. We stroll through the neighborhood, looking at the heritage houses and commenting on the architecture.

This morning Doctor John and I discussed a specialist who treats patients with malnutrition. He is worried about my sixty-pound weight loss and thinks I should consult with a physician in that field. What he says makes sense, and I have agreed to the appointment.

The shelves of the tiny shop are cluttered with pattern books, embroidery threads, and wools of every color. I am in craft heaven. The scarf I've been knitting has grown slowly and is now the ultimate length for winter wear. It's time to discover another craft to fill the long hours. As we leaf through the catalogues for ideas, I explain to Mom that Hardanger (a form of needlepoint) has always interested me, because it resembles Victorian handiwork. I purchase a few supplies for the small pillow, smug in the fact I've made this trip without my wheelchair, and with just a short breather on the shop sofa.

Mom performs the Healing Touch tonight, her energy, much more potent than Akash's, pulsing through my body in powerful waves. When she finishes, I experience an unpleasant sensation, as if electricity has passed through me.

**May 27**

"Which way did your mother spin your chakras at the end of your session?" Akash asks.

"She spun all of them the same way, counterclockwise," I reply.

Akash gasps as I explain what happened last night during my Healing Touch session. "How do you feel?"

I explain that I have felt agitated ever since my session.

"Heather, have your Mom redo the Healing Touch to make certain the chakras are spinning clockwise. Once your Mom learns the correct technique, you will find that the sessions benefit you both.

Healing Touch helps not only the person who is ill, but the healer as well."

It's strange that Akash should mention the benefits to the healer. Mom and I had been talking this morning about the way the treatment has provided some relief for her sore shoulder; Akash had no knowledge of our conversation. She is right, as Mom and I have just completed another session, and I feel immensely better once the chakras are spinning in the correct direction.

I have phoned Debra to compare experiences again. This time I'm less terrified of long term treatment with Formula.

"Heather, it took me three months to work up to three hundred calories." Talking with her gives me confidence in my progress on a day I reached the six hundred calorie mark, using the slower method of increase.

**May 28**

Lois has replied to my letter, revealing the thoughts and emotions of someone who has been trapped in a weakened body much longer than I have. A kindred spirit, she writes of a life tragically altered by an inexplicable malady which started with flu-like symptoms. Much of what she writes reflects my thoughts and experiences.

"I know the frustration of it all—you just want to scream. It's like being in a small prison cell day after day, week after week, month after month. I call it a 'living hell'."

## CHAPTER 10

# THE KEYS

The ring holds keys of many shapes and sizes. Each one unlocks a crucial passage of the labyrinth. Am I clever enough to use this valuable gift?

# The Toxic Labyrinth

## June 1

I inch down the stairs, tears welling in my eyes with each painful movement. Although daily walks have become an integral part of my recovery, today my symptoms have reappeared, and the strength required to reach the path by the healing ocean waters eludes me.

"We don't have to go if you are not well," Mom says.

I'm determined. These walks are helping me regain my independence. I can't allow myself to slip back.

The waves wash gently against the sand. Leaning heavily on Mom's arm, my shoulders bent and rounded from the ravages of weight loss and malnutrition, I perform the shuffle of the invalid elderly, the walk I have seen so often on the hospital wards. From the path, I can observe children building sand castles and running along the beach. Their energy makes me envious, but spurs me on. One foot in front of the other. Baby steps.

An envelope of materials has arrived from The Clinic. Sifting through the information, I realize there is much to learn about the facility, and the effect common chemicals have on our bodily functions.

## June 2

The white coating on my tongue seems to persist no matter what I do. Has the continuous sipping of Formula throughout the day caused an infection in my mouth? Even though I'm brushing my teeth every four hours to combat this, I may need to be more vigilant about my oral hygiene.

## June 3

The burning in my stomach and mouth has increased, and one by one, symptoms are returning. When I review my daily records, I notice a strange cause and effect relationship. I am brushing my teeth more frequently, and at the same time, my symptoms have escalated. Is the toothpaste causing this change?

## June 5

By eliminating the toothpaste, I have reduced the symptoms and rid my mouth of the white coating. Kathy's warnings about personal care products and chemicals in our environment may need to be considered more carefully. Are my symptoms more than just allergic reactions?

It's a small hill, but a hill, nevertheless. Several days ago walking this route would have been impossible. Today I stride unaided toward the crest. When Mom and I are almost there, we have to turn back, not on my account, but because it is starting to rain.

Day twenty-four drinking Formula and no food; this new course of action appears to be working.

## June 6

Mom has suggested I phone the toothpaste manufacturer for a list of ingredients. We have become very cautions about labels on packaged products, a wariness that is well founded. When we were researching allergies, we discovered there are substances used in the manufacturing process that are not required to be listed on the label. In addition, many personal care products do not list even basic ingredients. My toothpaste is one of them.

For competitive reasons, the company representative will not reveal the ingredients so I try another tactic. Reading from a list of toxic ingredients, I ask about the presence of each one in this particular brand. She confirms or denies the inclusion of each named ingredient. Hanging up the phone, I'm satisfied that I have made the correct decision to eliminate toothpaste.

# The Toxic Labyrinth

**June 7**

Another hallmark day. Not only am I walking unaided, I'm walking unescorted, careful to keep the apartment in view at all times. Because my symptoms no longer catch me unaware, I don't require companionship for this adventure.

Mom and I have spent hours discussing my progress, which she compares to the development of an infant. Drinking Formula and learning to walk without assistance are the first stages. She is convinced that my body will soon accept solid foods and has even wagered money I will achieve this goal by October. Today I resemble a toddler and exhibit a little independence by venturing from the apartment, yet I still keep the parent in view.

Later, on my visit to Doctor John, the wheelchair is nowhere in evidence. The staff are amazed at my vigor and comment that the sparkle has returned to my eyes. Still concerned about my sixty-pound weight loss, Doctor John emphasizes the importance of my appointment with the internist who specializes in malnutrition.

In relating my history to Doctor Sam, the internist, I focus on the joint pain rather than neurological symptoms. Experience has taught me to be cagey when presenting information to the medical world. Joint pain is safe from psychiatric investigation.

Although knowledgeable about food intolerance, Doctor Sam does not understand why I've lost all tolerance to food. He suggests hospitalization for a series of tests, but I refuse; no more hospitalizations for me. We agree that, if I'm not eating within six months, I must consider another route. Even though he is worried about my nutrition, he does not consider me anorexic. No one as committed to eating and the continuous drinking of the foul tasting Formula could be labeled anorexic. For now, I must build on the nine hundred calories I've attained. Concerned about the monthly cost of Formula, he offers to write a letter to help me obtain financial assistance, but requires the confirmation of special testing for this. I decline his offer, because I will not submit to any more testing. Somehow, we'll manage the cost.

It's strange how life moves in circles. Doctor John had phoned the coordinator of the anorexia clinic, a psychiatrist, to discuss my case. It was the coordinator who had confirmed I was not anorexic and had suggested an appointment with Doctor Sam. I'm certain the coordinator did not recognized my name. But a number of years ago, I nursed his daughter who had cancer.

**June 8**

There is still reason for concern because my weight has not stabilized. A pharmacist, whom I've know for some time, is educating me about TPN, in case this procedure becomes necessary. After confirming there are preparations for sensitive people like me, he tells me of a patient who has become allergic to everything and lives in the hospital; at least I have not reached that point. I vow to keep fighting, to keep drinking Formula: anything to avoid being incarcerated again in a hospital ward.

I am angry that Doctor Joe has suggested psychiatric counseling to help me cope with this chronic illness. The upsetting part is not the suggestion, but rather the stigma of the word 'psychiatrist'. To change the focus of the conversation, I mention the sessions with my counselor which Doctor Joe seconds as a wise decision. Leaning back in his chair, he paints a picture of my future life, one filled with children and normality. How can I even think of that goal when I've had so many setbacks? In my world, the future is only one day at a time.

The information from The Clinic has alerted me to the effects of chemicals in the environment. Each day I watch the newspapers for articles about environmental toxins and their role in the breakdown of our health. Mom says that once the press is reporting daily on this type of problem, it has reached dangerous levels.

# The Toxic Labyrinth

**June 9**

The session with Akash is exhilarating, but unnerving. My mind generates colors—red and purple, brilliant in their intensity. I drift off, as if in a dream. Mom is part of the dream. Although I can't see her face, I can hear her voice. Who is she calling? I can't hear the names. Intuitively I know she is calling to her grandchildren. Is Doctor Joe right that the future may be filled with children and good health?

**June 10**

A miracle of sorts. Don is home, I'm not in the hospital, and we have the apartment to ourselves for the weekend. Enjoying the company of each other, we wile away the hours without having to anticipate a crisis at every moment.

"Don, I know I'm making progress. I've started dreaming again, something I haven't done for months. I still mourn for the time lost, the months of my life I can never regain."

"Even if it takes longer than we anticipate until you are fully recovered, what are one or two years of crisis in our lives compared to forty good years together?"

Words meant to comfort are diminished by the fear of regression, my constant companion. If only I could be certain that I've turned the corner, that the forty good years will become a reality.

**June 15**

Don spins the chakras under Akash's supervision. Like Mom and me, he is willing to try anything to improve my health. The hives on my throat are making me uncomfortable and he is spinning the chakras, performing the Healing Touch to open the energy fields. To relieve the cold in my left hand, Akash demonstrates the way Don can move his hand over mine in a clockwise direction. The movement creates a shock which courses up my shoulder and through my ear, releasing the cold as it travels. Today's session is no different from the others. After each session, my symptoms reappear for a time, lower back and flank pain especially. As the day progresses, my body realigns and the pain disappears.

Another letter from Lois, this one filled with the poetry she has been writing to cope with her illness. Tucked among the papers is a poem she has dedicated to me. I read her words, words which vividly express my thoughts.

*Prisoner in My Body*
*(to Heather)*

*I am a prisoner in my body*
*and a sick body at that.*
*I long to be free, to sail away*
*but each day holds me back.*

*On one side, and out the door*
*are many wonderful things-*
*The blue sky, the sun, the grass.*
*Oh, Lord, just give me wings!*

*People walk about their ways,*
*I hear the things they do.*
*I remember a time, seems long ago,*
*that I was about things, too.*

*I am a prisoner in my body,*
*I cannot follow them.*
*I look at the ceiling, then close my eyes,*
*I let this world grow dim.*

# The Toxic Labyrinth

*On the other side, and out the door*
*are other wonderful things-*
*The blue sky, eternal sky.*
*Oh, Lord, here I have wings!*

*I read God's Word and it takes me far,*
*my spirit is so free.*
*I walk and talk with One who cares*
*Oh, Lord, I am with Thee!*

*A prisoner in my body*
*I am between two doors.*
*Jesus set my spirit free,*
*and there my spirit soars.*

*Lois (Millar) Cooke*

## June 19

My eye is swollen. The burning and shaking are constant. Can I manage the long flight to the Clinic? Don says I don't have to make the trip if it is too taxing. But each stage of my recovery has been guided by an inexplicable force, which I dare not ignore. This facility is another component in my healing process, one that will play a major part in my rebirth.

Large jugs of Formula and distilled water, my sustenance for the day, form a major part of our carry-on luggage. Thankfully we are flying first class. As my symptoms escalate with each hour in the air, the vision in one eye becomes totally impaired from the swelling, and the burning in my chest is extremely uncomfortable. Don holds me, fearing I may pass out.

# The Keys

What a relief to be off the plane and inside the hotel room. As Don spins the chakras, he comments that all my energy fields are blocked. With each movement of his hands, my body greedily transfers their energy to replace my depleted reserves.

## June 20

We're not prepared for the colorless, barren apartment that will be our home for the next ten days. Two mismatched army cots, covered with cotton bedding, stand alone on the stark tile of the bedroom. The living room is sparsely furnished with everything metal: a park bench, table, four chairs, a lamp, and an air filter that hums in the corner. Is this apartment an image of my future? Am I condemned forever to a Spartan existence, devoid of any warmth and color?

A cotton shower curtain provides the only softness in a bathroom covered from floor to ceiling in ceramic tiles. The bright lights harshly illuminate my frame, revealing the tautness of skin over bone. Gingerly, I step into the enamel tub and lower my hips onto the towel placed strategically to prevent my skin from bruising. The bathtub used to be associated with warmth and comfort, but now only reminds me of the depletion of my body.

A shopping trip to the mall. Size one. My new clothes attest to my sixty-pound weight loss. Was it just last Christmas I had to settle for size fourteen? I must be suffering from jet lag and lack of calories. The mall is making me confused. The apartment building coordinator had mentioned the mall might make me ill. Do all the new arrivals suffer from jet lag at first?

## June 21

No perfumes, no hair sprays, no food, no plastics—the long list of forbidden items on the door warns us that we are entering a purified zone for the critically sensitive. Don and I are glad we prepared for

# The Toxic Labyrinth

the strictness of The Clinic by pre-ordering special personal care products. Will they consider my Formula, which I still have to drink continuously throughout the day, food?

The large waiting room is simple, and like our apartment, furnished with metal chairs and the ubiquitous air filter. This is obviously not the opulence one usually finds in a private clinic.

Patients, many with cotton masks hanging from their necks, converse in quiet tones while waiting their turn. The dynamics of the room suddenly change when a woman enters and sits down. Several of the patients quickly put on their masks in response to what she is wearing. This action makes me realize how much I have to learn about subtle irritants that elicit this type of response. But I relax about my own situation, confident that the causes for my illness are not similar to what I am observing.

The size of The Clinic becomes more apparent, when I move from the waiting room past the numerous examining rooms. Here again, metal and tile prevail. Only a small square of cotton towel breaks the bleak austerity of each examining room. Staff and patients rush through the corridor, making rapid decisions in the midst of chaos. Like a child on the first day of kindergarten, I try to assimilate my surroundings, convinced I am the only one who is bewildered.

Doctor Pete is writing while I relate my story. His empathetic and soft spoken manner assure me he will listen as I confide my entire history. I have discovered that most of the staff at The Clinic have been ill at some time because of exposure to environmental toxins, and Doctor Pete is no exception. I won't have to defend my sanity here.

He examines me, his skillful hands performing a karate chop motion over my body. Thank goodness I'm better than I was a month ago, when I couldn't bear any pressure on my skin.

"What you are, and have been experiencing is very real," says Doctor Pete, assessing my history. "I see lots of nurses in The Clinic who have problems as a result of working with chemotherapy. I'm relieved that your bone marrow tests show no signs of cancer. But we do require a number of blood tests."

He explains that he wants to make certain that my body is not making antibodies against itself, that there are no proteins in my urine, and that my body is harboring no chemicals. I balk at the suggestion of skin testing to determine what I can eat, even though the organic food extract, used in this procedure, is prepared especially for The Clinic. No more injections for me. Doctor Pete quietly says I can take my time to find out more about this testing. I will think about the food testing for a while.

The next step is a visit to the dietitian. She wants me to test for foods before designing my personal nutritional program, but I still I am wary of this procedure.

"What are my chances of gaining back my tolerance to food?" I ask. She replies that sometimes patients regain tolerance to only two or three foods.

Once we are out of earshot, Don remarks, "Well, isn't she Suzy Sunshine."

Don maneuvers the car along the interstate.

"How are you feeling?" he asks.

"My chest is tight and I'm beginning to feel unwell," I reply.

"My eyes are burning. Let's find a better place to spend our afternoon." With that remark, Don pulls into a park in a residential area. The improvement in my chest is almost immediate. This incident triggers my memory. How many times had I experienced shortness of breath and chest pain while driving on the interstate highways in San Antonio and Memphis? When Don and I spent a weekend of sightseeing in the countryside, the tightness in my chest improved immediately.

Tonight as I down the last drop of Formula, I hold up the jar and shout, "Hooray!" Twelve hundred calories. How far removed I am from the feeding tube in May.

# The Toxic Labyrinth

## June 22

Yes, here I sit on the edge of the metal stool in the food testing room. With Don watching from the waiting room, I feel like the child who wants the parent nearby in case anything bad happens.

Last night, I phoned Mom to ask her opinion about the food testing. After mulling over my question, she gave her opinion. "The testing is done with very minute amounts of food in surroundings where people observe and record your reactions. Professionals will be there to assist you if a particular food causes a problem. It will be much easier, if you can find even two or three safe foods before you start eating, so you don't have to experiment by yourself." Her argument made sense, and I have agreed to try the food testing.

Are people really allergic to salt? They must be, since the first test is to determine my reaction to saline. This is good way to build up my confidence. Saline is not likely to cause a reaction. Other than the vitamin IV, I've never had any trouble with IVs which contain saline as the primary ingredient.

The next test is for histamine, an important measurement for the whole testing process. Apparently the tester has to determine whether my immune system is working and at what level. If I have no reaction to histamine, this means my immune system is not functioning. Knowing the level of my immune function is crucial in case I react to a certain food, and the tester has to bring me out of the reaction.

However, my test for seratonin produces an instantaneous reaction. Sweat runs down my face, pain encircles my chest and stabs at my stomach while the room spins, pulling me deeper into a void of blackness. I steel myself to keep from fainting. The tester keeps injecting me to find my level and end the reaction, all the while insisting I should be in the testing room for patients who are extremely ill. Silently, I keep urging my body to fall in line. I don't want to be in that restrictive testing room where my Formula would be banned. Finally, after what seems to be an eternity, my body functions as it should.

The testing sessions have exhausted me. Don, excited about his day of research, wants to regale me with stories related by patients in the waiting room and show me the new books filled with information on environmental poisoning. The patient conversations reveal that many have been poisoned by pesticides, and the gravity of their conditions has had a dramatic impact on Don.

"I think we should go to shopping at the organic grocery store," he says.

"Don, I'm not ready to eat, yet. I don't even know what I can eat."

"I don't want to shop for you. I want to shop for me. I want to buy food that hasn't been treated with chemicals," he replies.

I smile to myself. Interesting words from a man who used to ridicule organic food and recycling. Now, after a few days of listening to horror stories in the waiting room, he has converted his thinking without any prodding from me.

**June 23**

With my notebook open, I'm ready to record any reactions during the first day of food testing. The tester has warned that after I experience three reactions, the testing should stop. How do I gauge what is a true food reaction and what is a symptom? I'm still experiencing symptoms, but at a much lower level than before. Will they interfere with my observations?

I've chosen foods that tend to be low on the allergy list: lamb, broccoli, millet, beets, turkey, squash, carrot, watermelon, chicken, and rabbit. Only beets and turkey have given me a slight skin reaction so far. What a great way to build up a list of foods.

# The Toxic Labyrinth

A red weal spreads quickly over my arm, proof that rabbit is not a food of choice. The tester injects histamine to clear the reaction, which signals the end of today's food testing.

I've collapsed on the floor outside the testing room. Don leans over me, concerned that we should be informing someone of my condition. I assure him that the reaction will pass.

After we return to the apartment, the barrage of symptoms continues. Don phones The Clinic. Our orders are to return for a drink to reduce the reactions.

To augment the drink, Don has administered the Healing Touch and is now walking me around the apartment. God, I feel like I'm going to pass out. Numbness envelops my body. My hands are swollen, unable to close. Blackness closes in and for a moment my vision is completely impaired. Finally, the symptoms recede after two more sessions and much more walking. No food testing tomorrow. Enough of that for a while.

**June 24**

Apparently, I'm not identifying my reactions to food precisely. By the time I had tested for the rabbit, my body had been building up reactions from some of the other foods. I have discovered the importance of observing both the internal and external or skin reactions. Don and I have agreed I will stop testing food after the first reaction, no matter how small it is.

The barren simplicity of the apartment serves to illustrates the difference between a chemically free environment and the toxins my body faces on the outside. Inside the apartment, my body manifests few symptoms, but once I leave this protective environment, things change. The effects of the pollutants and other chemical assaults make me appreciate the healing process created by the sterile environment of The Clinic and the apartment. But this discovery also frightens me. Will I become the woman in the bubble?

Looking out the window and wishing for the pleasures of outdoors, I remember Donny one of my cancer patients in the bone marrow transplant unit. Restricted to the isolation room of the ward for most of his two-year life, his suffering typified the pain and emptiness many of my patients experienced. Nose pressed against the glass of his prison, he would watch us at the nursing station, his dark eyes pleading for release. Like me, he couldn't leave that room without wearing his mask. No, I can't take control of my future, if I think about such things. Baby steps. Think about baby steps.

Don says The Clinic reminds him of a Club Med for the chemically sensitive, accommodating people from many different countries whose lives are governed by a schedule of daily activities. For me the place is more. Finally, I'm meeting people who are like me or worse, people who validate that my experiences are not 'all in my head'.

**June 26**

Melissa is visiting for the weekend. A nursing buddy from my 'traveler' days, she introduced me to the Hispanic culture by teaching me to speak a little Spanish. With her coaching, I related more easily to my Hispanic patients and their families.

We have spent the last hour shopping in the outdoor mall. Most of the stores did not bother me, except for the potpourri shop which brought on the familiar numbness. Now, sitting on the patio of the Mexican restaurant, I smell the aroma from the red peppers. This is one food which is high on my avoidance list. Even handling them, when I cook for Don, causes a reaction. I don't want to spoil my time with Melissa, but I hope she will eat her lunch quickly, so we can leave.

Using Don as a guinea pig, I demonstrate the power of the chakras to Melissa, who is fascinated by the power of Healing Touch. Don's chakras swing wide, demonstrating the force of his energy fields which are powerful enough to impede the functions of a wind up watch.

**June 27**

Because Don and I have agreed that I will leave after experiencing the first reaction, the food testing room feels less threatening today. The tester injects the organic-apple food extract under the skin of my right arm. Hives appear on my left hand. Strange reaction. Injection on the right side, hives on the left. Does this relate to the predominance of symptoms on my left side throughout my illness? Whatever the reason for this phenomenon, I'm not here to figure out why; one reaction means it's time to leave.

Sandra, the massage therapist, is poised, beautiful, and stylish. Her vivacious personality radiates energy into the room, while she explains that deep lymphatic massage is necessary to release the toxic chemicals stored in my tissues. She warns that when the body releases these poisons after the massage, it is common for patients to feel ill for a period of time. Regardless of the short term effects, my reading has shown how important physical manipulation of the tissues is for recovery.

Later, Becky, one of the patients, recounts her story while we move the game markers toward the finish line. "It's been so difficult for me since I got sick. The ventilation system in my school put chemicals into the air which circulated through my classroom. Lots of us got really sick after that. Even the teachers got sick. The school trustees kept saying there was no problem. Finally, my Mom brought someone in to inspect the school and prove that the ventilation system had been installed the wrong way.

"The doctors back home don't believe me when I tell them I get sick in the mall. I even have asthma attacks when I read the newspaper. I couldn't go to school all last year, because I was too sick.

# The Keys

"My art has always been important to me. While I was sick, it was the only thing I had the energy to do. Now I'm bored with it. I want to be outside. I want to play with my friends."

Becky is echoing my thoughts, this twelve-year old girl who has to overcome the same obstacles as I do.

## June 28

Sandra was correct. Although I felt ill for a few hours after yesterday's massage, I feel great tonight.

Despite its stark simplicity, this place gives me the courage to think about the future. The radio is playing our favorite country music, songs which evoke memories of dancing and parties; songs I haven't wanted to hear for a long time. I couldn't bear the thought that such an important part of my life was over. Laughing and joking at the metal table, Don and I pretend our apartment is a bar.

"Can I get you a drink? he asks.

"Bring me a Formula light," I quip.

Don bows, takes my hand and asks me to dance. As we sway to the rhythm of the song, he whispers in my ear, "I promised you would dance again."

## June 29

The list of tasks, all to be accomplished before we leave The Clinic tomorrow, seems endless. My new lifestyle demands a commitment to making my environment more friendly, free from the toxic chemicals that have played a major role in my illness. Our apartment is filled with a bedroom air filter, natural cotton bedding and clothing, non-toxic personal care products and cleaning supplies, and books. All of these items must fit into our already burgeoning luggage. We have arranged another visit to The Clinic for six weeks, the next time

# The Toxic Labyrinth

Don is home. The progress I have made in the last ten days is amazing, but so much more is possible.

## June 30

On the drive back from the airport, Mom comments on the improvement in my appearance. Although I'm still thin, my weight has stabilized, and I have managed to gain a couple of pounds.

Mom's apartment is causing my symptoms to reappear. Even with the air filter, I'm better outdoors than inside. There is nothing we can do to alter this situation, other than stripping the rooms bare of carpets and furniture. Something has to be done quickly about our living arrangements, before Don leaves for Nigeria on Monday.

## July 1 and July 2

The hunt for an apartment is in full swing. Although I'm skeptical about finding a place, Don is very optimistic. We man the phones, armed with a list of our requirements: hardwood or tile floors, no pets, and no pesticides. In error, I assumed that apartment buildings in northern climates are free of pesticides. Unfortunately, a city by-law requires apartments to be pesticided. One option remains, a suite in a private house. Even though Mom's apartment bothers me, at least it's free from pesticides. The time is ticking. What can we do in two days?

The tiny basement suite, at the exorbitant rent of six hundred and ninety dollars a month, can be ours immediately. Looking at the mold on the windows, soiled carpets over a tile floor, decrepit furniture, and mediocre appliances, I wish this was not our only choice.

The owners are departing on a short holiday in a few hours, forcing us to make an immediate decision. Sitting in the car, we discuss the apartment. Don is enthusiastic and assures me, with a little ingenuity, improvements can be made. I don't share his enthusiasm, but finally, give in as we have no alternative.

Although the rugs and furniture have vanished, the apartment is too moldy for me to enter. Through the window, I watch Don vigorously scrub the tile with our non toxic cleaning products, determined, with each stroke of the brush, to make this place a refuge to continue my healing process.

### July 3

As I walk through the door, my chest constricts with each step. After all his work, how can I tell Don the apartment is not safe for me? When I place the charcoal mask over my face, the tightness in my chest starts to subside. This may be the way I can help Don wash the windows and walls. Don puts on his mask and together we begin the arduous task of removing mold and grime.

We survey our handiwork. Everything sparkles. New wood and recently painted shelves have been covered with tin foil to eliminate any toxic fumes, and small fans circulate the air. A water filter is installed in the shower and the unit for the kitchen sink has been ordered. From the corner, the air filter emits an assuring hum. Hopefully, within four days, this metal box, which removes over one hundred toxins from the air, will complete the job and make this place habitable for me.

### July 4

Making the bedroom less toxic is the most important step in my quest for better health. The metal bed on the showroom floor is perfect, particularly since I won't have to worry about assembling it.

Pieces of the white metal tubing are scattered across the floor. Regardless of how they maneuvered, the delivery men couldn't bring the bed through the door without taking it apart. I can't deal with this.

# The Toxic Labyrinth

Ordinarily I would be able to cope with such a trivial matter. These days, there are no extra energy reserves to deal with anything but remaining alive. I sit on the floor, surrounded by this mess, and cry.

## July 7

Tentatively, I enter the apartment without my mask. Inhaling deeply, I hope the filter has cleaned the air. No reaction. My habitat is austere, without warmth, but livable.

My research indicates that by law most mattresses are treated with pesticides. The one I have purchased is specially created from organic cotton and without any toxic treatment, but emits a pungent odor which pervades the apartment. Was it sprayed with pesticides by mistake? Although it is midnight, Dad suggests to be safe, we should remove it. I cry as we lug the burden out of the apartment, into the car, and drive it the couple of miles to Mom's apartment, where we leave it to air out by her living room window. Is there anything more that can go wrong this week?

## July 10

How long has it been since I've cooked food? A pot, a dish, some cutlery, what else do I need to accomplish this exciting task? Nothing is going to deter me from eating my first meal—that is if a quarter teaspoon of food can be considered a meal—not even the tough skin of the acorn squash.

I touch the squash with my tongue. A taste sensation unlike anything I've ever known bursts through my being. Mom says food is a symbol for me, one of returning to the normal world. When I complete my ritual, the exhilaration from my accomplishment confirms her theory.

**July 11**

My bedroom is complete with the cotton mattress. Mom has returned, and after smelling the mattress, has declared the scent to be raw cotton, not pesticides.

My sense of smell is attuned to those places that are not safe for me. As I continue to eliminate toxins from my body, those senses that were dulled have become sharper. Hardware stores, lumberyards, malls, and drug stores are not friendly places. The chemicals contained in the products and in the construction of the buildings provoke the return of symptoms that have faded in the past few weeks.

**July 14**

Although my apartment is healing my body, I find it depresses my spirit. Only one small space, a window seat where I spend most of my time, is inviting. The rest of the place is dark and cold, even in the heat of the day.

A tap on the window. Mom has come to rescue me from my dungeon. I put down the sweater I'm knitting and join her outside for our regular evening walk and conversation. We have been reading any materials and books we can find on the effects of toxins and environmental pollution. Most of the time, our discussions center around what we have learned.

Tonight, after returning from our walk, I reflect on the progress we have made in determining the causes for my illness. What was once a maze of unrelated events has become less of a mystery.

My life, until now, has been an example of the way people are exposed to chemicals without knowing this is happening. Most of us are unaware of the impact that the common chemicals, the so-called friendly additions to our twentieth century life style, are having

# The Toxic Labyrinth

on our health. What a different course my illness would have taken if I had understood this relationship.

The world revolves around speed and convenience, and this is contrary to the way our bodies function. Many different chemicals are used to manufacture or treat the products which fill our homes, cars, and workplaces, and thousands of new ones are being added to this burgeoning group each year. We have to be extremely devious and well informed to keep chemical exposure to a minimum, and reduce the toxic overload on our bodies.

Some of these chemicals are very unstable and continuously move from the product into the air we breathe. Outgassing is a term commonly used to describe this movement. I recall my experiences in the shopping malls, drugstores, and clothing shops which left me dizzy and confused. Malls are toxic warehouses, poorly ventilated and full of items using chemicals as part of the manufacturing or packaging process. When the chemicals outgass into the air, they have no place to go except into the lungs of shoppers, like me, and store employees.

Not only are we breathing and eating these chemicals, we are also absorbing them by using personal care products. The toothpaste I no longer use contained formaldehyde and ammonia. Now, to make certain that the ingredients are safe, any product I use on my skin, teeth or hair has to be labeled.

So many people are unaware, like I was, of the danger to their health. How many people are experiencing the first stages of chemical overload: a flu that doesn't disappear, chronic fatigue, heightened sensitivity to smells. My problem didn't begin in Memphis; it has been with me for years. By the time I collapsed, my body was overloaded with chemicals and couldn't cope.

Allergies seem to play a big part. All of the people I met at The Clinic suffer from allergies that make them more susceptible to chemicals and pollutants. Their bodies already identify certain foods, dusts, pollens, or other factors as intolerable substances. In addition to this, when they are constantly exposed to common chemicals in their living and working environments, the body shows signs of distress and signals an overload. I'm a good example of what can happen.

My stomach aches in high school were the beginning of my decline. Because they were a regular part of my life, I learned to ignore them. At first they were probably caused by allergies, but later, chemicals came into play. When I was at The Clinic, I started to piece together my history. Hanging in the waiting room was a chart illustrating the most dangerous environmental chemicals, and chlorine was at the top of this list. That chart made me think about the way my stomach aches increased during the last two years in high school. At that time, I was spending at least fifteen hours a week swimming and working as a lifeguard at the indoor pool.

The next few years did little to improve my health. Like most university students, my diet was less than nutritious. I never thought I had time to eat properly. To make matters worse, I was so concerned about my weight, I would go without meals. Sometimes, I just drank coffee and chewed bubble gum. Even when I did eat, the residence meals were often high in fat and simple carbohydrates, and the vegetables overcooked.

Seven years ago, when I was misdiagnosed with Crohn's disease, I had been working as a lifeguard for the summer. By that time, my body was not as healthy as when I was in high school. Five years of poor nutrition at university had taken its toll. The only reason I recovered from that first attack of environmental toxins was because of a change in life style.

After the diagnosis, I quit drinking coffee and alcohol. Then, I moved to Vancouver where I rented an older apartment with hardwood floors. The state of my finances dictated minimum furnishings and decor. After a few months, I stopped taking the medication prescribed for Crohn's disease. With all of these changes, I was living a relatively chemical free existence by accident. The flu-

# The Toxic Labyrinth

like feeling disappeared, my stomach aches lessened, and I had few health related problems for a while. Because my stomach aches did not disappear completely, I know some of my symptoms were caused by allergies. The reason I haven't had any problems with my stomach recently is that I'm drinking only Formula.

After I started feeling better, I reverted to some of my old ways. I drank coffee and alcohol again, although I was probably eating a little better than I did in university. My stomach problems increased with that change.

My stomach aches eased again during my second contract in New Orleans, when I changed my diet. However, my apartment was a toxic nightmare. It had no ventilation and was sprayed regularly for cockroaches. Mom was ill for two months after she visited me for a week. Thankfully, I spent most of my time in Don's spacious house.

San Antonio was the place where my health really deteriorated. I changed my diet again, this time to beef, pasta, and lots of cheese. It was my second assignment on a pediatric cancer ward. I moved there in August and by November I had developed bleeding gums and asthma. I celebrated my birthday in February with a flu I couldn't shake for three months.

By the time I had moved to San Antonio, I had been working with chemotherapy for three years. Six months into my contract, I couldn't work with certain types of this treatment. I would become short of breath and experience a crushing feeling in my chest. The other nurses on the ward would have to administer some of my patient chemotherapy treatments for me. During that time, I noticed the numbness in my left leg, and I was always tired which I attributed to the twelve-hour shifts. Adding to my problems, the apartments in my building were sprayed twice a week with pesticides.

When I moved to Memphis, I felt tired and ill most of the time. The numbness and tingling I had experienced while driving on the interstate in San Antonio was even worse in Memphis. I began to develop claustrophobia, especially when driving through tunnels.

Flashing lights bothered my eyes, and I couldn't hold my gaze on anything for more than a few seconds. This lack of concentration also affected my driving.

After working an eight-hour shift and absorbing the chemicals circulating throughout the hospital, the exhaust from the interstate would overload me. To top off this toxic mixture, I would eat TV dinners packaged in plastic. By two o'clock in the morning, my body was trying to rid itself of all the chemicals I had encountered throughout the day. What is most alarming is that my life style was not much different from most of the single women I knew.

The fungal infection in my lung was probably developing in late August, and the shot to enhance my immune system in September was the 'last straw'. Although, we initially thought the infection was caused by a fungus found in the southwestern dessert, it may have been something as simple as yeast. In spite of the aggressive treatment with the fungal medication, there was an above normal level of yeast in my sputum even after the mass in my lung had disappeared. Of course the medication for the fungal infection and the 'die off' of the fungus added to my chemical overload.

I used to wonder why the testing made me so ill. Now the cause is clear. Each time chemicals were used in the procedure, the load on my body increased. The barium tests were the worst, because it stayed in my body for such a long time. Of course, it was not a prudent decision to take a laxative to alleviate the problem.

The fluid diets and IVs reduced the load on my body. Each time I was admitted to hospital or the emergency room, my body had a chance to rest and rid itself of some of the toxins before I started eating again or had another test. The length of my recovery periods varied, depending on the substances that had entered my body prior to the escalation of my symptoms.

Many times in the past year, I have been poisoned without knowing the cause. My afternoon at the beauty salon, the plastic fumes from the oxygen mask in the ambulance, our special weekend

# The Toxic Labyrinth

in the renovated hotel, and the recirculated air in the airplane are just a few.

With each piece of information, I realize the far reaching effects the environment has on our health. But there is much more to learn about those poisons that are slowly disabling or killing us.

## July 15 to July 18

Paula scolds me for not calling, and I explain that until now, I haven't wanted to spend time with friends. There was nothing to discuss, nothing in my life except my illness. I amuse her with stories about my experimentation with food and my excitement about eating even though most of the foods are not common fare. But she is into fitness and health and knows about millet and squash.

Perfumes and bath oils are prettily displayed on shelves with antiques and lace trimmed doilies. What should I buy for Carol's birthday? Just a few minutes inside the store before my eyes burn and my hands are numb to the elbows. In the past I wore perfume, collected a new scent each time I traveled. Is this the way it will be for the rest of my life—confined to a cold, colorless apartment with none of the touches that give me pleasure?

The sun glances through the needles of the pine trees. Walking through the ancient stand of trees, Bob and I discuss his newest engineering project. How could I have predicted that our friendship would remain so solid over the years? During my first year in university, Bob spent innumerable hours teaching me the theory of physics and the wonders of coffee as a study necessity. I have been ever grateful for the physics lessons, much less so for the coffee habit. As we walk deeper into the trees, my concentration wanders. Words break through the fog in my mind, chaff from a conversation that makes no sense. Usually I can cover my confusion, but I have to admit to Bob I'm having a problem. This frightens me. Am I regressing?

The ceiling of the megastore reaches twenty feet above the concrete floor. It is stark, devoid of carpets, and furnished with metal and wood, making it possible for me to concentrate long enough to pick out a filing cabinet. Mom and I measure and compare. What will fit into the small space in the apartment? I must house all my papers inside a metal cabinet to avoid the effects of the chemicals in the ink and paper.

I haven't walked the streets of Chinatown since last December. Mom and I trudge up the hill toward the center of the shopping district. Rain threatens from low clouds slung like hammocks over the city. Buses pass, spewing exhaust into the faces of pedestrians. Stores with doors open to attract customers line the street. A variety of aromas wafts from each, mingling as they penetrate the air around us. Ripe vegetables and mounds of garbage waiting to be collected add to the overpowering mixture. The setting is becoming too much for my body to handle. We pass a shop stocked with herbal medicines, their pungent odors overwhelming and acrid. My head is spinning and the sense of confusion is disorienting. We must leave, while I can still make it back to the car. Each of these occurrences forcefully emphasizes what I have been reading about toxins and chemical overload. What would I have done by myself in this same situation?

**July 20**

Mom and I are out for our usual evening stroll. Walking along, I hear the comforting clunk of the glass jars filled with Formula and water that I carry in the blue bag slung over my shoulder. Not too long ago, the smell and taste of Formula was nauseating. Now the liquid represents life and what little future I dare think about. Many of our conversations focus on what I perceive as my lack of future, and this evening is no exception.

# The Toxic Labyrinth

"Mom, I have no identity any more. I used to be a nurse, someone with a career and promise for the future. What does my future hold now? I can't go back to nursing. If that was the only change it wouldn't be so bad. It's not just the problem of a career change. I have to give up so much. Am I destined to live in a place devoid of any comfort or color? Travel, dining out, working in different locations was so much a part of my life. Now I can't do any of that.

"When I was sick the present was unbearable, thinking about the past was depressing, and, at that time, there was no future. Now I can think about the future, but I there is no future out there for me."

"Heather, I don't believe it will be as bleak as you say. If you think about where you've been, you have accomplished so much in such a short space of time. In May, you were attached to a feeding tube. Your body needs time to heal.

"Once you build up your body, it will be able to handle more of a chemical load than it can right now. You will always have to be careful. Everyone should, if we expect to remain healthy. Now that you are vigilant about your nutrition and keeping your home environment chemically free, your horizons will expand again."

"But what am I going to do? I want to get back to work. I hate being a financial burden on everyone. What will I do if I can't work in the hospital?"

"Don't worry about your career. Your experience this past year is similar to taking a doctorate in environmental illness. What better knowledge can you have than to have been the laboratory rat. There is a future out there for you. It will come to us as you recover. For now, just concentrate on getting better. The rest will follow in good time."

"Time. I've been sick for a year, Mom. All of this has taken too much time already."

"Remember the body follows an exponential pattern in both sickness and health. Your body succumbed slowly for many years.

When it became overloaded it spiraled down at a much faster rate, giving the appearance of an immediate collapse rather than a downward trend.

"That same pattern will be in effect as you recover. The recovery will be slow at first, and you must have patience with that pace. Once you build your nutrition to a certain point, the body will respond exponentially upward. You'll find that suddenly, many of your functions and abilities will return."

"I worry that my body will backslide. My symptoms are not as severe as they were, but they are changing. That scares me. I was used to the old symptoms. The familiar isn't as frightening."

"We know your body has stored a lot of the chemicals it couldn't unload, didn't have the energy to unload. Now as it gets rid of these chemicals your symptoms will change. It's part of the pattern. I think, as your body heals, it's sending out different signals than it did when you were very ill."

"Yes, I guess I'm going through a rebirth and I have to achieve each goal one step at a time. It's been so hard this past year. I'm just afraid to plan for the future in case I'm disappointed again."

**July 29**

I carry my washing up the stairs to Mom's laundry room, proof of the ongoing return of my strength and energy. Each day I add another achievement to my growing list which now includes driving the car, shopping, long walks, and lengthy visits to Mom's apartment.

Doctor Pete wants me to continue drinking Formula until I have gained at least twenty-five pounds and can eat a balanced diet. I don't mind. It's strange how a person adjusts. At first, I hated the taste of the Formula, and now it represents my passport to the future.

# The Toxic Labyrinth

**July 30**

Kevin and I laugh at the small bowl of organic squash sitting before me at the restaurant. Yes, I had to bring it with me. It is my link to normal eating, and I cherish this moment.

A rainbow of color showers from the sky. I lie on the blanket, looking toward the heavens, watching the intricate patterns of the fireworks as they magically transform the blackness of the night. Kevin, Carol, and Ron share this wonderment with me. We are surrounded by young and old alike, enjoying the atmosphere created by fireworks moving to the accompaniment of music. The Symphony of Fire, a Vancouver summer ritual, is a toast to my new beginning.

**CHAPTER 11**

# EXIT VICTORIOUS

My hands reach out grasping the warmth from the sun. I celebrate victory.

# The Toxic Labyrinth

**August 1**

Tomorrow I leave for a six-week stay at The Clinic. We all agree that my recovery will proceed more quickly, if I avail myself of this assistance. Unfortunately, an illness caused by toxins in the environment is not covered under any medical plan, and I worry about the escalating costs. The financial drain has taken it toll.

One more problem in this year of problems. Don is supposed to meet me at The Clinic, but there is unrest in Nigeria. With the workers on strike, some of the airlines will not land in the country. If his replacement cannot fly in, Don may not be able to leave this month. When I undergo treatment, Don's support, gives me the courage to 'go the extra mile'. Although we have arranged for Rhonda to stay with me in late August, I do need his help during the first few weeks.

**August 2**

It's 5 a.m., and Dad is waiting to drive me to the airport, but my keys are nowhere to be found. I hope this dilemma isn't an indication of what the rest of the day may bring.

A six quart jar of Formula and three jars of distilled water make me a target for the customs officer, who asks me to open my bag for inspection. This man, guardian of the United States from terrorists and criminals, does not comprehend the reason for my jars. He looks through my passport. The TC permit left over from my working days as a 'traveler' arouses suspicion.

"Do you intend to work in the United States?" he asks.

I don't want to get into the complications of clinics and treatments. "No," I reply, "I work in Canada."

"Where do you work?"

Caught in a lie, I name my former hospital. Satisfied, he lets me enter.

# Exit Victorious

"Heather Millar, please report to the Delta Airlines counter." Why is the loudspeaker in the airport lounge blaring my name? I'm just here to change planes. Has something happened to Don, to Mom? Maybe customs has found out I'm not really working and is going to deport me. With my heart racing, I slowly make my way to the counter to find that the airline is putting me on another flight.

The receptionist is sorry, but my private apartment is not ready. Unfortunately, the current tenants want to stay longer and refuse to move. Apologizing for the inconvenience, she asks if I will share with a couple, until another place becomes available. The woman is very ill and will likely be in the hospital. Her husband spends most of his time with his wife, returning to the apartment for the evening. I'm scared. If Don doesn't get out of Africa, I may have to fend for myself with some strange man. What can I do? Surrounded by bags and jars, tired from my twelve-hour flight, I agree.

My fears vanish when a kind and gentle person answers the door.

"Come on in," says Mike. "Marsha's in the other room. I'll introduce you." When Marsha takes my hand and welcomes me into her life, I know I have found a kindred soul.

Mom is on the phone. "Heather, Don sent me a note on Internet to say he has left Nigeria and will be there on Friday."

The fear that Don might be in danger, a fear that I did not dare admit even to myself, is released in a flood of tears. A wonderful ending to a rather hectic day.

**August 3**

Doctor Pete hands me the test results from my previous visit. The first paper lists the forty-two amino acids, essential building blocks of the body; I appear to be missing nineteen. The second paper contains the more frightening fact that my body is making antibodies to attack

# The Toxic Labyrinth

my gut. I ask Doctor Pete why this would be happening and he says that medical science has no explanation. It is miraculous that I'm alive and as healthy as I am. The next step is to replenish my amino acids as quickly as possible. Doctor Pete has given me some capsules, but I'm afraid of taking such a concentrated amount at one time. What if I have a reaction?

Back at the apartment, the jar of Formula on the table gives me an idea. I open the capsule and poor the contents into the liquid, a solution that will satisfy both Doctor Pete and me.

Marsha enters my bedroom and asks how I feel. Knowing that I'm apprehensive about taking the amino acid capsule, she asks me to wake her if I have any problems during the night. Her kindness has changed my mind about roommates. Having someone close at hand, who understands the loneliness and terror of the night, is what I need right now.

**August 4**

How does one discuss bowel movements and constipation delicately? I guess there is really no way. Those who suffer from a bowel disorder know how wonderful the feeling is when the bowel starts working again. Today is a banner day for me; one more part of my body is functioning normally.

Marsha has warned me that walking to the grocery store can be hazardous at rush hour, but I'm feeling energetic today and the distance is not that great. Just a few minutes into my walk, and I realize she is right. I'm not as well as I think. The fumes from the exhaust are making me confused, and I must turn back before I lose my sense of direction.

**August 5**

My world is complete. Don and his pickup truck, our vehicle of transport for the next few weeks, have arrived via Memphis.

Sandra, the massage therapist, puts the paddles against my feet, explaining that the light electrical current may help my body detoxify. Though I'm not secure about wires connecting me to an electrical current, at least no one is injecting me with medication. The deep lymphatic massage which follows is not relaxing. To draw out the toxins from my body, Sandra's practiced hands push deep into the tissues, a motion causing my mind to become hazy and confused. The confusion escalates until, finally, I lose the ability to speak. But this altered state doesn't frighten me any more. I know each session helps to release more of the poisons making me ill.

**August 6**

Blisters in my mouth. Burning in my hands and feet. Evidence that my body is dumping more toxic waste.

I tried lettuce today, reacted, and left the testing room immediately. I'm still maintaining my rule of one food reaction per day.

**August 7**

How many people have heard of amaranth? Well, I can eat it. There is so much we don't know about the body. Why can I eat amaranth and not a simple food like lettuce?

Before I left for The Clinic, Akash gave me the name of someone in this city who practices Healing Touch. I have discussed the benefits of my sessions with Marsha, and she is willing to try the technique.

# The Toxic Labyrinth

One might assume that those who practice Healing Touch represent the weird and occult in our society, but this image is false. Andrea, like most of her fellow practitioners, is a nurse, an ordinary woman who could be my mother. She begins the session without asking any questions. Moving her hands over my body, she says, "I have a guardian angel who works with me when I heal. While I work, I always ask the guardian angel what each person needs to speed the healing process. You are the first person I don't have to tell to drink more water."

I smile to myself thinking about the quantities of Formula and distilled water I drink each day.

"I can't advise you to do anything differently. You are doing all the right things. Life is becoming more enjoyable each day. This enjoyment is reflected in your ability to see colors as you saw them in childhood, vibrant and vivid."

How could she know about the colors? I hadn't told anyone, even Mom, about my renewed ability to see colors as my body heals.

"The taste of food will take on a life of its own. You will experience an explosion of new tastes. Food will form a new dimension in your life.

"Whenever you feel ill, stand in the room and hold out your arms. Turn clockwise. Stretching exercises will also help your body heal."

I have learned not to prejudge any piece of information that comes my way these days. If I wait and listen, the meaning of her comments will eventually be revealed.

Marsha and I discuss the evening. As she did with me, Andrea has voiced thoughts and feelings that Marsha has held inside.

### August 8

Marsha has confided that last night was the first time in a very long while that her sleep was filled with dreams, instead of nightmares.

Whatever the power of Healing Touch, it certainly assists the body to harmonize with the universe.

With each visit to Sandra my periods of sickness after the deep lymphatic massage decrease. This is especially true, when I visit her regularly. Today, she manipulates my back muscles. "Heather, your shoulders are rounded from lying in bed for so many months. I want you to start stretching exercises to strengthen your back muscles and correct this." How interesting that she and Andrea have similar ideas about what will help with my recovery.

My vow to never have another IV has to be broken. My body needs to be replenished with the amino acids it lacks. The IV room will soon become the place where I will spend most of my days. Now that Don has arrived, I can start to build up my body. His presence is important in case I react to this treatment.

The IV room, stark and bare, contains metal chairs and stretchers with simple cotton covers. We are very sick, those of us who are here. The room must be free from anything that might cause us to react.

There is both good and bad about the atmosphere. It is good that everyone in the room understands why I'm here. There are no doubts in their minds that I truly belong to this group, a group that has no label. Even though we refer to our condition as environmental illness, this is not a definitive label; rather we represent those who collectively have a myriad of symptoms, undefined by any medical text. Yet, we *are* ill and we *want* to heal.

The build up process is slow. For the first few days, I must spend eight hours in this room, so my body can adjust to the infusion of amino acids. Rushing the process is as dangerous as no treatment. Too much too soon may allow the body to detoxify rapidly, making me extremely ill.

I listen to the sound of voices echoing from metal walls that have contained the agony of many lives halted by the body's inability to deal with our new world. It is frightening to hear the stories of new or renovated houses, pesticides, unhealthy work environments, leaking silicone breast implants, and hair dyes, from normal people who have entered the world of the abnormal.

I'm afraid of the IV. My experiences until now have done nothing to raise my confidence in any solution entering my body by means of a needle. The old timers reassure me that shortly this procedure will be routine.

The fluid in IV bottle is almost drained. As the day has progressed the burning in my hands, feet, and mouth has disappeared. Maybe my friends are right, and this treatment will help to heal my body.

Don walks me around the apartment to keep me from fainting. The flu-like feeling is back; my brain is enveloped in fog. Is this what detoxification is all about? Reacting and detoxification are so similar. The symptoms I have experienced for so long were merely warnings that my body emitted to signal toxic overload. In an effort to detoxify, it unloaded the toxins through whatever passage it could. Until now, the process was too massive for my body to handle without assistance. Hopefully, by reducing the toxic intake from the environment and building up my nutrition, I can supply the assistance my body needs.

The reactions have finally disappeared and I feel great. This process will be repeated many times in the next few weeks. The reactions don't frighten me, now that I know the cause.

**August 9**

I'm eating little bits of food. Like a prisoner, newly released from a concentration camp, my first contact with smells and tastes is powerful. For months, I have kept these sensations alive in my memory. Now, every so slowly, a little bit of reality is being introduced.

I look at my first foods squash, millet, chicken, and broccoli. Even with harmless foods, ones that cause no reaction, I must be careful to rotate my menu each day. I have devised a schedule: two days of safe foods plus Formula, a day when I try a new food and drink only Formula, and one day of Formula alone. It's difficult not to eat every day, but I must be vigilant. When I listen to my body, it clearly tells me to move with care.

Don says my skin tastes and smells acrid, like a chemical dump sight. Am I losing some of the toxins through my skin? This is quite possible since the skin is a major organ of the body.

Today I tested for buckwheat and peaches. Peaches have tested negative for now and I'm disappointed. But Don is philosophical about the whole process and says if I gain one food a day for six weeks, I will have over forty foods by the time I leave. I guess he's right. Still, I would like to eat peaches.

We have moved into our own apartment. Even though Marsha and Mike were great roommates, having our own space allows me the freedom to pace late at night without disturbing anyone but Don.

Waves lap against the shore, the bright patches of sunlight riding each crest like boats sailing into harbor. Stretched out on the sand, I reflect about the influence that water has had on this illness. Why am I so much more vital beside the water? Is it because I'm an Aquarius? For months my condition was characterized by an insatiable thirst. Does water assist the body in eliminating the toxins? Is that why Don can taste the chemicals in the sweat on my skin?

**August 10**

As the days pass, I am learning more about my reactions to food, facts that would have helped me during the first food tests. Had I known what to observe, I could have avoided the intense reaction to rabbit.

# The Toxic Labyrinth

My internal food reactions of spaciness, cramping of hands and feet, and shortness of breath are much more powerful than a skin reaction. Because they resemble milder versions of my original symptoms, I haven't related them to food. Now that I'm wiser, I can stop the testing before I build up too many adverse symptoms.

Each day my symptoms go through a subtle change, as if I'm ridding my body of toxic layers. As the layers are stripped away, the symptoms regress to earlier reactions, fleeting warning signs my body issued long before my collapse in Memphis.

"Take a back seat, Henry the Eighth," I laugh at the chicken bones scattered across the plate. I may not be able to eat many foods, but those I can, are finished down to the last morsel.

## August 12

Not one of my better days. I had a major reaction to alfalfa sprouts this morning and felt as if my chest was closing.

## August 13

Don has confined me to quarters, specifying that there will be no testing or food, just relaxation.

We've walked miles around the apartment while my body unloads. Symptoms have come in continuous waves throughout the day. Finally, evening has brought calm, a peace that I relish because it demonstrates my body's increasing ability to deal with the environment.

## August 14

I've persuaded Don to lift the ban on outdoor activities, so we can spend the day visiting local sights. Psychologically, I require contact with the world outside, even if it means dealing with the toxicity.

Although I expected to react on the freeway, insulated by my charcoal mask and the special air filter for the truck, I'm handling the day very well.

The Victorian village, a composite of restored houses and antique shops, is just what the doctor ordered. How lucky for me my interest lies with the old rather than the new. Many of the materials used to build the houses and furniture of the nineties contribute to the toxic overload.

## August 15

Small amounts of vitamin B and trace minerals now enter my body through the IV. Each day, as my nutritional level builds, I notice an increase in the amount of supplements and food my body can tolerate.

Licking the final remnants of the lamb chop from my fingers, I celebrate a minor indulgence of flavor and fat. These days not one crumb escapes unnoticed. And what about a bagel for dessert? It's made from millet flour, water, and sea salt, a packaged food created especially for people like me.

Listening to my body, and the commitment to my wellness regimen is paying dividends. My weight is increasing each day, and gone is the pallid and gaunt scarecrow that stared at me from the mirror only weeks ago.

## August 18

We lie in the IV room, walking wounded from every part of the world, veterans of the guerrilla war being waged by our environment. We swap stories, laugh, and give each other hope. I learn a great deal from my comrades, more than from the doctors, whose time is limited. There are too many of us, too few of them. Those patients who have been in the system for some time 'know the ropes'. I listen and commit their advice to memory. Most of them have taken a longer route than I have to arrive here. Thankfully, my family relentlessly pursued every avenue and were tenacious enough to find a solution quickly.

Many of us have common denominators. The largest group is comprised of nurses and teachers, who often are employed in the most toxic workplaces. All of us have a history of allergies and women, by far, are the majority. The enemy strikes those of us who are most vulnerable first.

We describe similar symptoms. Agitation and confusion when driving the car. Unusual sensitivity to smells. Numbness and tingling in our extremities. The inability to tolerate certain places, such as enclosed shopping malls and certain stores, unfriendly areas which can bring on bouts of claustrophobia and confusion. Most have lost tolerance to a number of foods, starting with alcohol and coffee, then moving to wheat, dairy, and beyond. Once food intolerance becomes part of the picture, we quickly spiral down, the lack of nutrition compromising our bodies even further.

**August 19**

Guacamole dip won't be on my menu for a while. Even on a day when I'm drinking only Formula, my reaction to the avocado is extremely violent and leaves a red weal on my skin and causes excruciating pain from my underarm to my waist.

Sandra explains that my lymph system extends over the region where I experienced the reaction to the avocado. When the body detoxifies, many patients complain about the upper chest area, and the back of the neck just under the curve of the head, key regions from which our bodies tend to detoxify or react. She goes on to explain that the body can release toxins at any time of the day.

At 4 a.m., something has jolted me awake, but I'm not certain what. As I shake Don, I try to form words, but nothing comes from my mouth. Don calls this reaction my 'fish thing' because I resemble a gold fish under water. I would be scared, if my grapevine from the IV room hadn't mentioned this tendency for 'morning sickness'. Since the body works at night to eliminate toxins, patients often wake up when the body starts to unload.

**August 20**

I have just said good-bye to Don, who has left for a week's visit with his family. Looking excitedly at the arrival monitor, I realize how much has happened since Rhonda's last visit with me in March. Although we have talked frequently on the phone, and she has brightened my days with humorous notes and letters, nothing is the same as having her with me.

Now that Don has left, I am responsible for the transportation. My first day of driving the truck on the interstate has me worried. Even with the mask and the filter insulating me from outside influences, there is a chance that the pollution may affect me. While Rhonda and I laugh about her experiences on the plane and my adventures at The Clinic, a slight haziness begins to impair my vision. Recognizing this advance warning, I turn off the interstate and return to the apartment using suburban streets.

**August 21**

Rhonda has a new title, 'Washer of the Grains'. I realize the dust from the grains causes shortness of breath. I could wash the grains with my mask on, but Rhonda has volunteered for the job.

How ironic that Rhonda would benefit from our discoveries about toxins and chemicals. It seems the chronic neck problem and arthritic joint pain she has suffered for the past five years could be caused by her exposure to the heavy pollutants in London, and her eating habits. Now, she is as interested as I am in improving her health.

Reading and planing the next phase of my recovery together, we learn more about nutrition, both in relation to foods and total body function. The current belief that our diet provides enough vital elements and nutrients is not backed by the facts. Environmental pollution, modern farming methods, and processing techniques are leaching many of the required elements from our foods. Rhonda and I cautiously add vitamin C. We will introduce supplements one at a time to, ensure that our bodies tolerate this new nutritional regimen.

**August 23**

Sitting in the testing room, we discuss our favorite topic, food. Heaven for us would be eating without restrictions. However, we are pragmatists and realize our lives will never again be unrestricted.

In comparison with some of my fellow patients, I appear the picture of health. Now that I am over the initial excitement of my first discoveries, I look at them and wonder what's in store for me. Will I recover, or am I destined to the fate of recurrent patient at this facility. This possibility resides in the terror zone of my mind.

Today I don't want to hear the stories; I want to concentrate on wellness, not sickness. I don't intend to return. There must be success stories of people who have returned to the normal world. Why are there no achievements on the wall, pictures of the graduates to give us all hope?

**August 25**

My right ankle is throbbing and my entire left side is numb. Andrea places her hands over me. "What side did you have you IV on?"

"My right side."

"Your left side is on a different frequency than your right. The energy on your left side is disturbed."

It is the numbness in my left side that her practiced hands are feeling, not the effects of the IV. As she performs polarity work on my body, the sensation is so strong that it feels as if the toxins are coursing through my body and releasing through the top of my head. I lie on the table, exhausted and sick. Andrea comments that this Healing Touch session was like plowing through mud.

"Heather, my guardian angels have given me a message for you. It's important that you treat yourself to something 'sweet'."

Mom and I discuss my Healing Touch session with Andrea.

"What could I get that's 'sweet', Mom. I can't eat fruit or candy. It doesn't make sense."

"If you wait, the meaning of this message will come to you," she replies.

**August 26**

Don has returned to Dallas. Once again our time together has been short and associated with my health. Hopefully, his next trip out will not be spent at any type of health facility.

Rhonda and I are unwell after picking up Don from the airport. Both of us are too sensitive to tolerate the interstate, the moldy truck, and the jet fumes at the airport.

Mom has phoned with some interesting news. "Heather, the house where your apartment is located has been sold."

"My landlords didn't say anything about selling the house. Don just left the apartment today. There was no for sale sign."

"Well it's there now. But I think I've solved your riddle. Andrea's reference was to 'suite' not 'sweet'. You know that you can't live in that basement suite in the winter. It will be too cold and damp. You will have to treat yourself to new living quarters."

# The Toxic Labyrinth

**August 27**

We are attending an exposition to entertain Melissa who is visiting again. Fascinated by the many displays, we roam through the aisles avoiding areas with strong scents or odors.

Following today's excursion, I have only a slight headache; I must be getting better. Even a week ago, I couldn't have tolerated the building or the displays.

**August 28**

To give Melissa a proper send-off, we are going out to a restaurant, one that I can spend time in because it has hardwood floors. Even though I can't participate in the ritual of food, I'm able to visit and enjoy the surroundings.

Once Melissa leaves, Don and I take Rhonda on a tour of the Victorian village. How much better I have become. Many of the shops that were intolerable on my first visit cause me no problem today. I have found the perfect antique piece to show Don, who has gone to eat at a small restaurant down the block. As I approach the large windows, there he is for all to see, head down, right hand scooping the banana split without pausing. Second sight alerts him to my advancing figure. Looking over the top of his glasses, he visibly gasps and protectively clutches his treat, like a small child caught in a dastardly act.

Rhonda has learned a hard lesson during the ride home: never travel using just the cotton covering for the mask. The charcoal filter is essential for protecting our bodies during these excursions down the interstate.

**August 30**

Watching the action in the waiting room has become a diversion from my daily routine. The hours I spend in The Clinic would be monotonous if it weren't for the interesting personalities who enter its doors.

The woman in the jean jacket, complaining loudly about her IV, has caught my attention. Her toughness and arrogance make me wary, and I avert my eyes, pretending to be busy with my own concerns. From the conversation, I gather she one of the patients who stay in special housing outside the city, because she can't tolerate the pollution. Today she is very unhappy that she has come to The Clinic only to find her IV has not been scheduled.

After each food test, I return to the waiting room to discuss the results with Rhonda, who has replaced Don as my anchor. Rhonda is talking with the woman in the jean jacket. What could she find in common with such a person? I turn back toward the testing room before they see me.

"You must be Heather," a voice says. "I'm Elaine. Your sister has told me so much about you."

I look around to see who has spoken to me. To my surprise, the soft, caring voice belongs to the woman in the jean jacket. Maybe I've been too hasty in my judgment. She and I chat like old friends, exchanging details of the circumstances that have brought us to The Clinic. She tells of working on a highway paving crew and breathing the toxic fumes of the asphalt. Over a period of years, this exposure has produced such brain fog and confusion that, at times, she appears inebriated. Calculating her movements around walls and doors has become necessary to avoid sudden impact and the resultant bruises.

When Elaine speaks of her fight for sanity and survival, the image of toughness melts away and her kind and gentle nature becomes evident. Does one ever learn not to judge a book by its cover?

# The Toxic Labyrinth

**September 2**

In the IV room I have met ordinary people with lives that have been put on hold, those who have had to fight against being labeled 'crazy', because no real label exists for our condition. Each of them lives in a world centered around the pursuit of wellness. What is our future? I am not certain whether it was more terrifying when I thought I was alone, or now when I see the ever increasing numbers of people who are just like me.

Naomi, a beautiful spirit with a body emaciated from her long illness, is fighting the ravages of a badly ventilated office. Although she looks older than Mom, this is not unusual as most of the patients age prematurely. But when Naomi speaks, the image of chronic illness falls away, and the fiery spark that has kept her going emerges to light the room. We both drink Formula every day, our bond with each other. For her the IVs are important because during the last year she has been able to tolerate only three foods. Nevertheless, those three foods are important to her independence, and she intends to keep eating them. Naomi has a routine. Unable to eat in the IV room, she has to cap her IV when she leaves to eat. The stainless steel needles, made from a metal the patients can tolerate, are unstable. This, plus unhealthy veins, causes the needles to work loose. Naomi's trips in and out of the IV room make it necessary to restart her IV several times a day. In spite of this setback, she loves to laugh, her love of life inspiring those of us who sit close to her. She has been through so much, yet her spirit is unconquerable.

Jenny and I have the common bond of nursing and working with chemotherapy. But Jenny's body has been subjected to even more toxic chemicals from silicone breast implants that leaked and grew fungus. The first indication of a problem was her loss of vocabulary, which eventually led to memory loss. Recalling names, dates and events, through the fog that surrounds her mind, has become an impossibility. Her speech and motor coordination resemble someone trying to appear sober. Notes written in large letters plaster the walls of her apartment, reminders of routine tasks that cannot be forgotten. Full of life and fight, Jenny works each day to exercise her mind, to relearn those common tasks and simple words that most of us take for granted.

There are a few men at The Clinic, but the women by far outnumber them. Although the women are seemingly more vulnerable to environmental toxins, the men are also afflicted, but are restricted by society's image of toughness and often wait longer to seek assistance. Women console each other and form protective bonds to offer support. Men are left to drift in a singular void and internalize their thoughts and fears, a situation which isolates them further from friends and family. Afraid to be labeled as 'crazy' they suffer in silence.

Kyle typifies the male who is caught in this trap. He remembers, as a child, having difficulties with the smell of solvents when he visited his dad's shop. Now, he suffers with brain fog from working with general anesthetic. He and I often discuss the effects of anesthetic, especially on women who experience problems after childbirth or some other medical procedure requiring anesthetic.

## September 5

Rhonda and I walk around the lake, the ever-present masks shielding us from the pollution. These masks, protection from the excesses of our world of convenience, set us apart. Passers-by look at us with a mixture of derision and fear. Are we contagious? No we are the future. Our walk is an agreeable break from the demanding schedule of our wellness program: days consumed with shopping for organic food, cooking, IVs, food testing, reading, and massage therapy. Getting well has become an exhausting process.

We discuss Lois' arrival at The Clinic. Although Lois and I have corresponded, our meeting a few days ago at the airport was our

# The Toxic Labyrinth

first encounter in many years. A frail, thin woman greeted me from the wheelchair. Only a strong will and dominant spirit could have given this eighty-five pound body the resolve to make such a grueling journey. The atmosphere here has given Lois hope. She cried with relief, during her first visit with the doctor. No more pretending. No more trying to be what she is not.

**September 7**

I've decided to test my food orally, and today is my last day in the testing room. My inventory of edibles has increased so that I don't need to incur the expense of testing each new food. Sometimes the testing makes me ill, and it's time to set my own pace.

In some ways I will miss the testing room. The interesting mix of people. The trays of vials filled with organic extracts of common and exotic foods. The bin overflowing with disposable needles, at the end of the day.

The children are of special delight to me. How I miss my children. One of the biggest adjustments in my new life, will be finding another career. Nursing children has given me such pleasure, and finding a substitute will be difficult.

The children are most objective in their reactions to the food testing. Unlike adults, they have no preconceived ideas about reactions and results. Yoko quietly plays with her sister, and exchanging toys, they laugh with delight at the game. The tester injects Yoko with a food extract. Suddenly, she becomes a child possessed. Screaming in rage, she hits her sister on the head with the doll that minutes before was shared with such grace. Even from my vantage point across the room, I can see her swollen arm, the red welt spreading quickly from the point of injection.

She is just one of many who have reacted strangely within these walls. Personalities change in a matter of seconds from sunny to depressed or from quiet to violent. The staff keeps a ready supply of blankets to combat the chills and pervasive cold that overcome us as we try to unlock the mystery of our bodies.

**September 13**

Nothing is ever certain in my life these days. I have slowly introduced cabbage into my diet. Small amounts produced no reaction, so tonight I decided to eat a large plateful of this 'safe' food. I've miscalculated. The reaction is fierce and has awakened me with tingling in my back; burning in my hands, eyes, and chest; spasms in my left leg; and a headache that pounds incessantly. Have I set myself back?

**September 14**

I'm still reacting to the cabbage, and although the reactions are fewer, I don't want to make such a mistake again. Even water has produced symptoms these last few days.

**September 15**

Is anything in this life the way it first appears? How differently I view the apartment I once found stark and bleak. These surroundings now remind me of the people who have entered my life, filling my hours with warmth and humanity. Furniture and fixtures fade into the background, replaced by mental snapshots of friends and special times.

The surprise birthday party for Marsha. The group, masks hanging at the ready, make merry with a raw sweet potato topped by an unlit candle. The event has been catered with all our sensitivities in mind. No decorations (chemicals in the paper), no cooking (odors from the food), no lighted candle (the smoke goes without saying). To make the event a memorable one, we are left with the bare

# The Toxic Labyrinth

essentials, our wit and our wisdom.

The melt down in Elaine's apartment. Arriving home from a trip to the grocery store in the pickup, Rhonda, Elaine, and I pull up just in time to see a crowd massed outside the apartment complex. Curious, we inquire about the confusion. Smoke is billowing out of Elaine's apartment from the remainder of a baking project. Like many of us, Elaine has periods of brain fog and forgot to turn off the stove before she left. After a number of similar incidents, her apartment became uninhabitable, and she moved in with Rhonda and me.

Rhonda's video crusade. Armed with video camera, Rhonda and I fulfill a need to record the excesses of our environment. While posing in front of various backdrops, we attempt to film our message for the world. Unfortunately, the roar of the traffic and the efficiency of certain security guards, who usher us unceremoniously from the malls, make the task more daunting than we expect.

Quiet talks in the dark with Rhonda. Many nights we would lie together on the narrow cot, talking of our childhood and the different paths life has set for us. As the older sister, I was the caregiver, the one in charge, the one with the energy. Over the last few months, a reversal of roles has brought an equality and mutual respect to our relationship, more lasting than the illness which created the change.

## September 16

The plane climbs into the clouds, leaving the city behind. How dramatically my life has altered since that day in Memphis, a year ago, when Mrs. Phillips came briefly into my life. We were laughing and talking at the nurses' station. Some of the nurses from the next ward were relating stories about Mrs. Phillips, a mother of one of the children. According to them, she had an uncanny ability to read fortunes and make predictions.

"Of course she can read your fortunes. She watches and listens to you while you care for her child. I'll get her to read my fortune. She has never seen me. Let's see how accurate she is with my future." I would prove Mrs. Phillips was not what they thought.

I marched into the room, mustered my best poker face, and held out my hand. "I hear you read fortunes."

Without looking up, Mrs. Phillips took my left hand. "You are terribly ill. If you haven't been to a doctor, you must see one right away. There is a problem with your left hand. It seems to relate to arthritis.

"You are very unhappy with your situation. There is something you miss terribly that you can't find here. You will leave before Christmas. Three men will surround you and will be there for you. Shortly, you will receive a raise in pay."

At the time, I doubted the credibility of these predictions. Yes, the part about the raise in pay was true. That morning I had received a small increase on my pay check. But the rest, I ignored. Little did I realize how prophetic her words were.

**September 20**

A bulging file of cards and letters, mementos, and signposts of the past year, lies beside me. I pick up each missive, cherishing the thoughts and expressions of support from those who have believed in me.

A card from Denise brings back memories of my days as a 'traveler'. Denise was my recruiter who arranged the contracts. We had only met on the phone, until I had worked close to her office in Florida. Over the years, our friendship has grown. Her encouraging messages by mail and phone have brightened some of my darkest times.

I read through cards from Jessie and Gail, friends who have been part of my life for a long time. Although distance kept them from being with me, many times they have called at just the right time to give me my spirits a lift.

Christmas and birthday cards from my grandmothers express their wishes for my recovery. How difficult it must be for them to understand this twentieth century illness that has battered my body.

How many messages have I received from Don since this all began? Notes on the Internet. Cards mailed from his first airport stop while returning to Nigeria. These messages don't begin to tell the story of his complete devotion, or the hours spent with me trying to lessen the pain and perform small, comforting tasks. One of these tasks stands out in my mind, because of the patience and special skill it requires. Don loves my long hair and rejects any suggestion that I cut it. But chronic illness was not kind to my hair, and it often became snarled and knotted from rubbing against the pillow. Don would brush my hair, untangling a few strands at a time, until it fell over my shoulders in soft waves.

Not wanting to dwell any longer on the past, I replace the cards and letters in the file. It is time to go forward and define the future.

## September 28

A warm autumn breeze, the music to which the trees dance, embraces me as I walk with Mom through the park. The grace and beauty of their dance entices and captivates. Branches sway rhythmically back and forth raining leaves with each motion. The leaves, displaying the spectrum of fall in colors of red, orange, green, and brown, crunch beneath my feet. I feel an indescribable happiness to be part of this energy, an energy that has not been a part of my life for more than a year. For autumn is a subtle reminder of the beginning of my rebirth.

The sounds of spirited children playing a game of ball, echo from the park, their laughter reflecting our festive mood. Tonight we celebrate my new beginning and my journey of renewal.

Putting her arm through mine, Mom says, "There were times when I thought you would never be strong enough for me to do this. When we used to walk by the ocean with you holding on to my arm and shuffling beside me, I was terrified you would not make it. Or if you did, you would be disabled."

"You never let on that you were scared."

"If I had, you would have sensed my fear. I couldn't let you think there was anything but hope for your future."

"Mom, you know Akash and I were talking the other day. She said I had so little energy the first time she spun the chakras, I appeared to be close to death."

"When I practiced the Healing Touch I visualized you as a baby. You were healthy then and I wanted you to be able to start from that time. That's why I kept talking about baby steps."

"Do you remember in March when you spoke of one hundred and eighty days being a turning point? How prophetic that statement has turned out to be."

"Yes, there have been many signs along the way that have pointed us toward this end. Because we have actively sought a cure, we have been attuned to so much that might have eluded us had we resigned ourselves to the inevitable."

"Mom, now that I'm getting better, what can I do with my future? I'm so restricted. I can't go back to nursing. I have no identity, no purpose."

"We have discussed writing a book about our experience with environmental illness. I think it's important for us to tell your story."

"But I don't want to think about where I've been. It was so horrible. I just want to move on."

"Heather, this future you are looking for has been given to you over the past year. Ordinary people have to be alerted about what is happening to our world. The fact that you conquered environmental illness is very important. People have to be aware of the dangers and the practical changes they can make to avoid what has happened to you.

"It's even more important to make these changes to the environment for the children. We are raising them in a world that's becoming more toxic with each passing day. You saw for yourself the increasing incidence of lung problems and cancer in your pediatric patients."

"There were so many times this past year that I thought about my children. My life related to theirs in so many ways. But no one wanted to listen to me when I was ill. Why should they listen to me now?"

"They will listen. People are ready to listen."

Do I have the courage to look back into the past? Will one voice substantiate the reality of environmental illness?

As I look back at the children playing their game in the fading light, I wonder what is in store for them. What is their future? Yes, we have to write the book, if only for the children.

# INTO THE FUTURE

# The Toxic Labyrinth

The story of a life does not encompass only one year. However, in looking back, we often perceive one particular year as being more influential than others in the course of our lives. So it has been with Heather.

We felt compelled to leave our readers with more than just supposition about the months following Heather's return from The Clinic, and the epilogue highlights several events that have marked her progress, while the book was being written.

In October, Heather received test results indicating two chemicals BHC (benzene hexachloride) and HCB (hexachlorobenzene) were above acceptable levels. In fact, her levels of BHC were three times the acceptable level. These chemicals which affect the central nervous system played an important role in causing the neurological trauma that she experienced. Both chemicals are found in common household products and are used to treat agricultural products. However, Heather has diligently sought to improve her environment. This has escalated her recovery and resulted in the elimination of most of the chemical residues stored in her body.

On May 17th, when she was at her lowest point and attached to the feeding tube, Heather wrote out nine goals to keep her thoughts focused on recovery. In brackets are the results she has achieved.

GOALS MAY 17, 1994

1.    In six months I will be able to eat some foods. (She started eating July 10th.)

2.    In three months I will be able to take in 1500 calories a day. (In July she reached 1800 calories or six packages of Formula a day.)

3.   In one year I will be able to take in most calories with food. (By October, she had accomplished this. She still drank Formula for a few months after this to maximize her weight gain.)

4.   In three months I will be able to get up and have enough energy for a regular day. (By the time she returned from The Clinic in June, she could drive the car and was managing on her own.)

5.   I will not weigh less than 100 pounds. (Her weight stabilized at 102 pounds.)

6.   I will meet Doctor Brostoff in person. (Doctor Brostoff wrote the first book we bought on allergies and food intolerances. After reading it, we began to expand our search for information. Heather still hopes to meet him someday.)

7.   In three months I will be able to live independently. (She moved into her basement suite on July 7th.)

8.   I will make some forward progress without constantly regressing. (There was no regression in her condition after May 17th.)

9.   I will take my experience and help someone else. (This is her ongoing goal.)

The illness that threatened such devastation, has instead, lead to a whole new life style. Heather is now healthier and more energetic than she has been for years. Even the chronic stomach problems that she endured since her teens have disappeared. Along the way to optimal health, she has attained goals other than those she set out to accomplish in May.

In November she and Don found a new 'suite', a cozy home with hardwood floors and a view of the mountains. By December she had reintroduced many foods into her diet, had gained twenty-five pounds, and had included cycling and running in her leisure activities.

Don's time at home no longer revolves around Heather's illness. They have taken two vacations, including a month long trek back to the southern United States to bring back the remainder of their lives from Memphis. Although they had to travel equipped with filters and organic food, the trip was manageable. On her second trip in January, Heather had the opportunity to visit with her cousin Lois, who is ecstatic that she can now ride her exercise bike seven miles. (When Heather left The Clinic, Lois could walk slowly, but only with assistance.) On that trip Heather managed without her filter.

In January, Heather established a business to provide resources and assistance for those who are suffering from environmental illness. To celebrate her thirty-second birthday in February, she took her last drink of Formula. On February 9th, she added skiing to her list of leisure activities, and on that same evening she was able to join her friends at a nightclub. Her entry back into the 'normal' world was complete.

Unfortunately, Heather did not have the chance to share this last accomplishment with her Dad. On February 11th, he was killed when his plane crashed outside Modesta, California. Although his death has given Heather one more hurdle to conquer, she is comforted knowing he died 'living life to the fullest'.

Recalling events and reliving her experience for this book, has been one of the most difficult, yet rewarding accomplishments of Heather's life. Going back in time to a place from which she only wanted to escape was not easy. Her determination, to be a voice for those who suffer from environmental illness and an advocate to ensure a less toxic world for our children, has helped her achieve this goal.

$$\&$$

## CONCLUSION

# ARE YOU NEXT?

Although the chronicle of Heather's fight appears endless, that one year is considered a relatively short time in which to conquer environmental illness. Labeled as depressed or as hypochondriacs, many people suffer for years, never finding the cause of their chronic condition, and rely on ever-increasing amounts of medication to alleviate their symptoms.

Too often, the medical community resorts to a diagnosis of stress or anxiety when testing fails to indicate a definite cause for the symptoms a patient is experiencing. Although Heather was advised several times to take anti-depressants, we determined that this course was not an option, and a succession of events, during the early part of 1995 has proven this decision to be correct. Heather dealt with the trauma of her Dad's death, started her own business, weathered a spring with the highest pollen count in years, and fought off the flu. Most would agree that any one of these could be considered stressful, yet, in spite of these circumstances, Heather's health continued to improve.

Achieving good health is not easy because it demands sacrifice and sets limitations. But the fact that Heather's health is better than ever provides hope for those searching for a solution to illnesses for which there appears to be no cause. Although Heather's ultimate collapse was dramatic, her condition had deteriorated over a number of years. There is a mistaken idea that environmental illness results from one exposure to an excessive amount of a toxic substance. However, most individuals have been exposed for a number of years to common chemical toxins though their water, air, food, housing, workplace, and cleaning and personal products. Because this repeated exposure leads to chronic rather than acute symptoms, most of us do not make the connection.

We believe environmental illness is on the verge of becoming the epidemic of the twenty-first century and hope Heather's story has given you the impetus to evaluate your own situation.

Do you listen to your body when it shows signs of distress? Below is a checklist to determine whether you have some signs of sensitivity to the environment. The list is not exhaustive because this illness is unique to each person. Remember, always visit your doctor to eliminate any physical cause for symptoms you may be experiencing.

# YOUR TOXIC CHECKLIST

The items on the checklist are ones which we encounter daily. They are not listed in any particular order. If you check a number of the items on the list, you have reason for concern and should conduct further research.

## Places or Situations Where You May Feel Unwell

| | | | |
|---|---|---|---|
| ☐ | indoor shopping malls | ☐ | pharmacies/drug stores |
| ☐ | some clothing stores | ☐ | video/record stores |
| ☐ | perfume/potpourri shops | ☐ | dry cleaners |
| ☐ | lumberyards/paint stores | ☐ | photo studios |
| ☐ | printing shops | ☐ | photocopying shops |
| ☐ | interior design shops | ☐ | gas stations |
| ☐ | furniture refinishing shops | ☐ | hospitals |
| ☐ | energy efficient buildings | ☐ | new buildings |
| ☐ | newly renovated buildings | ☐ | smoke-filled rooms |
| ☐ | high traffic roads/intersections | ☐ | new cars |
| ☐ | swimming pools and hot tubs | ☐ | crowded rooms |
| ☐ | cloudy days | ☐ | hot days |

## Activities That May Make You Feel Unwell

| | | | |
|---|---|---|---|
| ☐ | driving | ☐ | exercise |
| ☐ | drinking alcohol | ☐ | drinking coffee |

# The Toxic Labyrinth

## Smells That May Make You Feel Unwell

- ☐ smoke (cigarette and wood)
- ☐ scented personal care products
- ☐ flowers
- ☐ burned food
- ☐ laundry detergents
- ☐ plastic
- ☐ car exhaust
- ☐ creosol
- ☐ asphalt
- ☐ newspapers & magazines
- ☐ copy machine/printer toner
- ☐ moth balls
- ☐ perfume
- ☐ pine scent
- ☐ some cooking odors
- ☐ strong spices & herbs
- ☐ cleaning products
- ☐ diesel exhaust
- ☐ gasoline
- ☐ burning oil
- ☐ paint
- ☐ fax paper
- ☐ moldy/musty objects
- ☐ chlorine

## Things That May Enter Your Body and Make You Feel Unwell

- ☐ skin creams
- ☐ certain foods
- ☐ testing dyes
- ☐ toothpaste
- ☐ medications

## Have You Experienced the Following?

- ☐ long term antibiotic use
- ☐ junk food diet
- ☐ silicone breast implants
- ☐ renovations to home/office
- ☐ installation of new carpet
- ☐ working in one of the toxic places listed above
- ☐ living in one of the toxic places listed above
- ☐ extensive medical testing where contrast dyes or medications have been used
- ☐ allergies
- ☐ fast food diet

&

# RESOURCES

# The Toxic Labyrinth

The following is a list of resources which we found valuable in our search for information on environmental illness.

## Health & Nutritional Information

Brostoff, Jonathan, M.D., Linda Gamlin. *The Complete Guide to Food Allergy and Intolerance.* New York: Crown Publishers, Inc., 1989.

Buist, Robert, Ph.D. *Food Chemical Sensitivity.* Garden City Park: Avery Publishing Group, Inc., 1988.

Crook, William G., M.D. *The Yeast Connection and the Woman.* Jackson: Professional Books, Inc., 1995.
Box 3246, Jackson TN 38303  Tel: (901) 423-8366

Crook, William G., M.D. *Chronic Fatigue Syndrome and the Yeast Connection.* Jackson: Professional Books, Inc., 1992.
Box 3246, Jackson TN 38303  Tel: (901) 423-8366

Crook, William G., M.D. *The Yeast Connection.* Jackson: Professional Books, Inc., Third Edition, 1994.
Box 3246, Jackson TN 38303  Tel: (901) 423-8366

Eades, Mary Dan, M.D. *The Doctor's Complete Guide to Vitamins and Minerals.* New York: Dell Publishing, 1994.

Joneja, Janice Vickerstaff, Ph.D., Leonard Bielory, M.D. *Understanding Allergy, Sensitivity & Immunity.* New Brunswick and London: Rutgers University Press, 1990.

Lieberman, Shari, Nancy Bruning. *The Real Vitamin & Mineral Book.* Garden City Park: Avery Publishing Group, Inc., 1990.

Randolph, Theron G., M.D., Ralph W. Moss, Ph.D. An *Alternative Approach to Allergies*. New York: Harper & Row, Publishers, 1990.

Rogers, Sherry A., M.D. *The Revised E.I. Syndrome*. Syracuse: Prestige Publishing, 1995.
Box 3161, Syracuse NY 13220  Tel: (800) 846-6687.

Rogers, Sherry A., M.D. *Wellness Against All Odds*. Syracuse: Prestige Publishing, 1994.
Box 3161, Syracuse NY 13220  Tel: (800) 846-6687.

Rogers, Sherry A., M.D. *Scientific Basis of Environmental Medicine*. Syracuse: Prestige Publishing, 1994.
Box 3161, Syracuse NY 13220  Tel: (800) 846-6687.

Rogers, Sherry A., M.D. *The Cure is in the Kitchen*. Syracuse: Prestige Publishing, 1991.
Box 3161, Syracuse NY 13220  Tel: (800) 846-6687.

Rogers, Sherry A., M.D. *Tired or Toxic?*. Syracuse: Prestige Publishing, 1990.
Box 3161, Syracuse NY 13220  Tel: (800) 846-6687.

Rogers, Sherry A., M.D. *You Are What You Ate*. Syracuse: Prestige Publishing, 1988.
Box 3161, Syracuse NY 13220  Tel: (800) 846-6687.

Rousseau, David, W.J. Rea, M.D., Jean Enwright. *Your Home, Your Health and Well-Being*. Vancouver, Canada: Hartley & Marks Ltd., 1989.

# The Toxic Labyrinth

## Product Information

Winter, Ruth, M.S. *A Consumer's Dictionary of Cosmetic Ingredients.* New York: Crown Trade Paperbacks, 1994.

## Cookbooks

Bumgarner, Marlene Anne. *The Book of Whole Grains.* New York: St. Martin's Press, 1986.

Crook, William G., M.D., Marjorie Hurt Jones, R.N. *The Yeast Connection Cookbook.* Jackson: Professional Books, Inc., 1989
Box 3246, Jackson TN 38303  Tel: (901) 423-8366

Martin, Jean Marie. *The All Natural Allergy Cookbook.* Madeira Park, Canada: Harbour Publishing, 1994.

Saltzman, Joanne. *Amazing Grains.* Tiburon: H.J Kramer Inc., 1990.

Saltzman, Joanne. *Romancing the Bean.* Tiburon: H.J Kramer Inc., 1993.

## Newsletters

AGES
(Advocacy Group for the Environmentally Sensitive)
1515 West 2nd Avenue
Vancouver  BC  V6J 5C5
Tel:    (604) 251-4697
Fax:    (604) 733-6506

Alternatives
(Washington Toxics Coalition)
4516 University Way NE
Seattle WA 98105
Tel:    (206) 632-1545
Fax:    (206) 632-8661

Canary News
1401 Judson Avenue
Evanston IL 60201

Environ
Wary Canary Press
P.O. Box 2204
Fort Collins CO 80522

New Perspectives
P.O. Box 1328
Renton WA 98057

The *New* Reactor
(Environmental Health Network)
P.O. Box 1155
Larkspur CA 94977

The Environmental Health Letter
Northeast Center for Environmental Medicine
P.O. Box 3161
Syracuse NY 13220
Tel:    (800) 846-6687

# The Toxic Labyrinth

<u>The Wary Canary</u>
Box 2204
Fort Collins CO 80522
Tel:    (303) 224-0083

# DISCLAIMER

*The Toxic Labyrinth* is intended as a biographical account of the stages of environmental illness and is not intended to give medical advice or other expert assistance in this field. The book is designed to provide information regarding the subject matter only.

The publisher believes the information presented should be made available to the public. However, the factors causing environmental illness and the attending symptoms are unique to each person, and it is important to check with a health professional to ascertain whether the condition is one which can be attributed to environmental toxins.

The authors and publisher disclaim responsibility for any adverse effects or consequences resulting from the use of any methods of treatment, procedures, or processes mentioned in this book.

# ABOUT THE AUTHORS

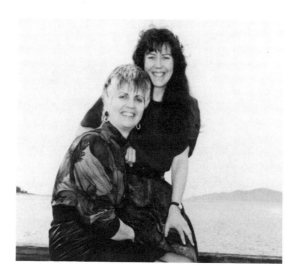

When Myrna and Heather Millar looked for a cause and effect relationship to explain Heather's illness, the evidence pointing to environmental toxins as the source of the problem became overwhelming. Further research and discussions with individuals, who also exhibit similar symptoms from exposure to environmental toxins, have revealed the magnitude of the threat this issue poses for the health of the general population, especially children.

These factors convinced the authors that telling Heather's story would provide a warning of the imminent and subtle danger of chemical toxins and a voice for those who suffer a condition rarely recognize by health care professionals.

Myrna Millar has a B.A. and B.Ed. from the University of Saskatchewan and a M.B.A. from the Harvard School of Business Administration. Heather Millar has a B.S.N. from the University of British Columbia and is a Registered Nurse in both Canada and the United States.